Slash your Weight & Trim your "Abs"

by John William Yee

Outgoing Press
Toronto

Copyright © 1998 John William Yee

All rights reserved. No part of this publication may be reproduced, stored in a retrieval system, or transmitted in any form or by any means, electronic, mechanical, photocopying, recording, or otherwise, without the written permission of the publisher except for brief passages by a reviewer for the purpose of a review, or in case of photocopying or other reprographic copying, a licence from CANCOPY (Canadian Copyright Licensing Agency), 6 Adelaide Street East, Suite 900, Toronto, Ontario M5C 1H6

Printed in Canada by University of Toronto Press Inc.,
5201 Dufferin Street,
North York, Ontario, Canada
M3H 5T8

Outgoing Press,
P.O. Box 45507,
747 Don Mills Road,
Don Mills, Ontario, Canada
M3C 3S4

Distributed in Canada by Husion House Publishing Limited,
36 Northline Road,
Toronto, Ontario, Canada
M4B 3E2
Phone: 1-416-285-6100 Fax: 1-416-285-1777

Distributed in the United States by Associated Publishers Group,
1501 County Hospital Road,
Nashville TN 37218
Phone: 1-800-327-5113 Fax: 1-615-254-2408

Cover photography by SuperStock, Montreal, Quebec
Photographic illustrations by John Yee and Scott Yee

Canadian Cataloguing in Publication Data

Yee, John William
    Slash your weight & trim your "abs"

ISBN 1-896212-06-9

1. Reducing exercises. 2. Abdominal exercises. I. Title. II. Title: Slash your weight and trim your "abs".

RA781.6.Y43 1998   646.7'5   C98-930395-0

*" Some men see things as they are and say, 'Why?'
I dream things that never were and say, 'Why not?' "*

— *George Bernard Shaw*

This book is designed to provide accurate and authoritative information with regards to the subject matter covered. It is sold with the understanding that the author, publisher, or distributors of this book shall have neither liability nor responsibility to any person or entity with respect to any loss or damage caused, or alleged to be caused, directly or indirectly by the information contained in this book. We recommend that you consult a licenced, professional health care provider for a check up before engaging in any exercise program.

Contents

    Introduction   7

1. A Horrible Thought   9
2. A Chance Meeting   11
3. What It's All About   14
4. Clarifying A Few Things First   19
5. The Intensity Factor   24
6. Sticking To It   29
7. The Catalyst   33
8. The Multiplier Effect   39
9. Getting Physical   44
10. A Prime Example   54
11. Playing The Part   62
12. Other Ways To Speed Things Up   66
13. Getting On Your Butt   71
14. The Good Old Ab Bench   77
15. Applying An External Load   85
16. Chalking It Up   90
17. Controlling Your Snacking Binges   93
18. A Bit About Crash Diets   99
19. Is It Necessary To Go All Out When Working Out?   104
20. The New (And Improved) You   114

    Afterword   118

    Charts   123

    Other Books By The Same Author   127

    Author's Bio   128

Introduction

Not too long ago, I was utterly shocked when I found that I had gained three inches around my waistline. Me of all people. I teach martial arts, and martial arts instructors are suppose to look lean and mean. Since I don't have a mean streak unless I manually switch it on, I depend a lot on the lean side whenever I make an appearance—especially in my classes for kids because they can see things that adults usually overlook.

If I tell them to do as I say and not as I do (or appear), it's not going to be effective. Besides, kids are impressionable; they will emulate me or my colleagues down to the last detail in words as well as in deeds (and sometimes even in appearance).

Moreover, I also compete. I had gained all that weight not only in the wrong places but also at the wrong time. My national championship competition was coming up, and I had my work cut out for me; in addition to brushing up on my techniques, I also had to lose a few pounds.

At first, I didn't think it was that difficult. I had faced harder challenges than that, but time was also an important factor. These days it is difficult to make a living just by teaching martial arts. I would often end up juggling two or three other projects at the same time, and I found I had trouble squeezing in some quality training—never mind setting up a separate program.

I thought that I would lose the inches from my waist as I workout, but that was not the case. I found that I had to do something fast. And you know…you can achieve amazing results sometimes when you're faced with a deadline.

I lost those those inches around my midsection in about two months. I was so excited about the effectiveness of this simple approach that I began to share my discovery with my selected group of students who were struggling with a weight problem—regardless of how hard they exercise. The next thing I knew, I had a special clientele, and I began offering private lessons.

The usual complaint from people who could not take my course was that it was hard to find time due to their other commitments. Believe me, I know how that feels.

That was when I decided to write this book. It contains all you all you need to know about "slashing your weight". As a bonus, I also combined it with techniques on how to "trim your abs" so that you can take it a step further. Yes, that's right. A set of "washboard abs" is definitely possible.

I will show you step by step on how to go about "slashing your weight and trimming your abs" in the following pages, and you can start this 2 in 1 program immediately in the convenience of your home. Besides the cost of this book, all you have to invest is 5 to 10 minutes a day.

To make it entertaining and easy to read, I have written it in the second person in a dialogue format. There is something magical about dialogue. You will see what I mean as it unfolds.

Enjoy,

John William Yee

1

A Horrible Thought

Suppose you suddenly realized that you had gained another 10 pounds. In other words, suppose you had done it to yourself again. You tried to restrain yourself during the holidays, but you couldn't. All that food, friends, and booze proved to be a deadly combination—as far as your weight was concerned.

You did not have such a problem the previous year; your weight would have adjusted automatically—not back to normal mind you, but back to whatever you had weighed before. Although it was above average, it was nothing to sweat over.

But that was back then. The scary thing that kept nagging away at you at the moment was that you might have to change your whole wardrobe.

"Maybe I should start buying clothes a size larger," you thought in anticipation. "No! No! No!" you said later. That was a horrible thought. It reminded you of cousin Jane who always did that. Whenever you saw her, it often made you wonder what came first: her oversized clothes or her increase in weight.

You decided for the umpteenth time that you should do some exercise. But you had this job that demanded a lot from you. By the time you got home, you just wanted to lay comatose on the couch for a couple of hours—never mind doing jumping jacks or rabbit hops around the living room. Just thinking about it was enough to stress you out, and you were already stressed out.

And dieting was also out of the question. You remembered what happened to cousin Jane who tried it. All that weight she had lost in such a short time—it was like a miracle. Then she decided to stop for awhile when she thought everything was almost back to normal. She had such high hopes, but it all came crashing down after she started putting the pounds back on.

But still—you wished that there was something you could do.

2

A Chance Meeting

Your wish was answered although you did not realize it when I stopped you at random. I did not know where all this was going myself, but I knew that I had to make a living. Business was slow, and that meant going out to make myself visible and start flogging it. I've been doing that for a few days now, and it was starting to get to me—especially after I just ran out of flyers and had to ad-lib. I was wondering if maybe mom was right. Maybe I should have stayed as a desk clerk at—

Several flashbacks suddenly jolted my memory. It was a rude awakening. I had to remind myself again as to who I was, what I was doing, why I was doing it, and why I had the nerve to stop you right in the middle of a busy intersection in the dead of winter.

"Excuse me, I'm conducting a survey. Which part of your body do you want to strengthen the most?"

"My midsection," you responded automatically.

"Are you doing anything about it?"

"I don't have time. Too busy at the office doing three different jobs at once. By the time I get home, I just want to relax."

"Would you be interested in a set of 'washboard abs'?"

"What's that?"

"It's fitness terminology. It refers to developing your abdomen until they ripple like a washboard."

"Didn't you hear me? I don't have time. Excuse me," you said as you tried to zigzag around me.

"But the routine will only take 5 to 10 minutes a day."

"A lot good that will do for my weight," you said without slowing down.

"That's also part of the course I'm offering," I said while trying to keep up with you. You were going at a decent pace; regardless of what anyone told you, I didn't think you had a weight problem.

"I thought this was just a survey."

"It is. It'll give me an idea of the level of interest before I offer it."

"It sounds too good to be true. A two for one deal?"

"Something like that."

"What sort of ridiculous price are you going to charge me?"

"Allow me to give you my card." It was the only reply I could think of after you made a dash towards the lineup that was quickly disappearing into the streetcar. "We can talk about it some more at your convenience. My studio is just a few blocks down from here."

"I've been working around this area for ten years, and I don't remember seeing a fitness studio."

"It's new. I just set up shop."

"I'll think about it," you said.

Most of my "surveys" usually ended on that note. But at least the interest was there.

3

What It's All About

"Hello?!" you echoed into the empty studio after you allowed a burst of cold air in behind you.

You stomped off the excess snow and huddled against the nearest radiator. Hot water pipes in an array of different sizes and shapes threaded across the ceiling and up and down the walls; it was an old building. My studio was at street level, and the windows along the length of it revealed the renovations I made. From the outside, it stood out like a sore thumb; but that was what I wanted—it was like free advertisement.

My office was around the corner, and I was deep in thought about the possibility of offering other types of courses once the weather improves. By then, people generally don't workout as much. I began to wonder if I was getting ahead of myself.

But that was how I came up with this new "Slash Your Weight and Trim Your Abs" program. I would never have thought about the idea if I had waited until people were ready for something different—something that offered convenience, a minimum of effort, maximum results, flexibility…

"Hello!" you called out again.

You took me by surprise since I was not expecting anyone until later in the afternoon. "Are you the person I talked to a couple of days ago?"

"Yeah, that's me."

"I'm glad you can make it."

"Listen, I have to get back to work in an hour," you made that clear before I could continue. "Can we make this quick?"

"Sure, let me show you around the place."

"We can do that later. Let's get right down to business."

"Here are some of the courses I offer," I said as I handed you a variety of brochures. You took a brief glance at them.

"I'm interested in the 'Slash Your Weight and Trim Your Abs' deal," you quickly decided.

"That's a popular one for people who are pressed for time."

"Yeah, I noticed that it's a one day session, and it's only for an hour."

"Apart from that, the actual routine only takes 5 to 10 minutes."

"Do I start with the weights? The treadmill? The stationary bike?" you pointed to each of them in turn.

"Actually, the first thing I want you to do is to change the way you think."

"Is this just some sort of behaviour modification technique?" you broke in. You sounded a bit disappointed.

"Not just on a conscious level but also subconscious. It also involves some physical exercises. You will do them daily, and it will only take 5 to 10 minutes. You don't have to go through an overall workout in addition to those exercises. That part is optional. But I do encourage you to become more active."

"That's it? Just 5 to 10 minutes?" you wanted to make sure.

"You can push it a bit more than that, but it's not necessary."

"Why?"

"When your physical commitment reinforces your mental commitment and vice versa, then that's sufficient. In a nutshell, that's what it's all about."

"What's the catch?" you asked.

"None. It primarily has to do with the *intensity* of your physical activity and not just the duration. Once you copy that *intensity* mentally, it will take you to a higher level.

Your *mental intensity* is like a catalyst. It will double or even triple the effect of your *physical intensity*. That's why I call it the *multiplier* and the phenomenon the *multiplier effect*.

A lot of people get caught up in the length of an exercise program to lose weight. Sometimes it works, and sometimes it doesn't. And even if it does work, you will be so drained from tearing across the country side or from heaving all sorts of weights and yanking away at pulleys—after putting in a hard day's work at the office—that you will be out of it for the rest of the evening.

The alternative I am offering you has been tested on various people: on a particular individual who I will introduce to you in a moment, on my students in my martial arts class, and on myself."

"So what exactly is this place? A fitness studio or a martial arts school?" you asked.

"It's both. I combine martial arts and fitness to give my clients a reason to exercise. Some don't mind sweating it out, but many of them cannot bear the thought of engaging in a vigorous routine for an hour when they could be doing something more productive."

"It's a waste of time," you sided with the latter.

"I try to compromise by offering a variety of approaches. If they want to get in shape plus accomplish something on the side at the same time, I have different classes for that besides martial arts. Others just want the sort of package that you're interested in: a one day seminar. They just want to know what to do, so that they can do it on their own at home."

"Developing my abs while I'm in the process of losing a few pounds..." you repeated to yourself.

"That's correct. It's actually a 2 for 1 package. You are going to lose some weight, and you are going to strengthen your abs—until they ripple. You are going to accomplish that in 2 stages:

In the first phase, you will commit yourself to 'slashing your weight and trimming your abs'. That's your mission statement. If you are out of shape due to excess fat, your primary objective during this period is to lose weight.

At the same time, however, you are developing your abs, and this goal can be just as important if you are slightly overweight. Keep reminding yourself that they are shaping up while you are shedding unwanted fat. You may not believe that it is happening at the same time if you can't see it, but curiosity here serves as an incentive for you press on—to uncover the flab and take a peek at what's underneath.

In the second phase, your next objective is to stabilize your weight once you got it down to a reasonable level. You might even start gaining a few pounds back within acceptable limits when you cut out the junk food, start eating right again, and build up some of your muscles.

How much definition your abs will actually reveal depends on how much fat you have 'slashed'. If it is a lot, there may be layers of loose skin around your waist. That is when you may want to resort to other types of exercises, like lifting weights, to firm up certain parts of your body to take up the slack before your friends can actually see the 'washboard' you have installed.

A lot of programs try to cram those two stages into one by skipping phase one and jumping right into phase two. But you cannot put the cart before the horse. Even a perfect set of abs cannot be seen behind layers of fat.

At the other extreme, some people become disillusioned when they lose weight without achieving the sort of waistline that they were hoping for. But if they were aware of the different stages of development that they have to go through, then they would have a different outlook."

"What about those who do not have a serious weight problem?" you asked with a hint that you might be included in that category.

"If you are already slim and the only problem you have is trying to get rid of a slight bulge on the sides and front of your abs, I still recommend that you start at phase one.

That slight blip is a sign of worse things to come. If you do not address the underlying problem of snacking or overeating, which you will also tackle during this phase, whatever benefits you gain will only be temporary."

"I don't think I have a gluttonous habit."

"You may not realize it at the moment. It always start as a minor and innocent activity. By the time it escalates, it becomes harder to correct. To make matters worse, you may not be aware of the habit.

The mental component of 'slashing your weight and trimming your abs' is just as important as your physical endeavours. That's why my program also consists of those two important aspects—as well as two phases."

4

Clarifying A Few Things First

You reflected on what I said so far. "It sounds simple enough."

"Well that is the thing about clear thinking these days. When you are constantly bombarded with megatons of information everytime you turn on the TV, with the promoter of one gut-busting product discrediting another, it is hard enough trying to distinguish the trees from the forest—never mind getting a glimpse of what's on the other side. To throw some light on this confusion, it would help if the viewer knows what he or she wants. Is it losing weight? A trimmed waistline? Washboard abs? Or all three?"

"The answer is obvious. I want to get my money's worth."

"If it's all three, then you have to realize something if you are overweight: you have to go through different stages of development. You cannot see rock hard abs without losing some weight first.
But this does not mean that those activities do not take place at the same time. In other words, my program will start the *process* of losing weight and strengthening your abs."

"The *process*?"

"You are not going to see a complete change all at once. There is no frog-prince effect. You are not going to wake up one day and find that you became a totally different person. Although the *process* takes place at the same time, it will not reveal those results at the same time. And you should also be aware that the *process* takes place gradually.

But the producers of some of those exercising gadgets for your abs—or 'Devices', as I will call them from now on—will often give you the illusion that you will undergo an instant change without going through different stages of development."

"And they seem to imply that when they bring out this gorgeous gal and handsome looking guy with the rock hard abs," you said when you thought about it.

"In most cases, you cannot even start the *process* of both losing weight and tightening your midsection by relying strictly on their Devices. Most of them are not designed for losing weight. They are mainly intended for building 'body mass'. There is a difference."

"So you are saying that your method offers 'toning' as well as building 'body mass'?"

"Those are the sort of results you will end up with. Because of this 2 in 1 effect, which is what slashing your weight and trimming your abs is all about, it will save you time. You do not have to engaging in an 'aerobic activity' like jogging or swimming one day to lose weight and in a 'resistance activity' like pumping weights the next day to build bulk."

"I used to jog. After I stopped for about a month, I found that I gained a few inches around my waist even though my diet is the same."

"Some people have this problem. They are fit and trim only when they are engaged in their aerobic activity. Once they stop for whatever reason, even for a couple of weeks or so, they will start to gain weight."

"Why is that?"

"There are a lot of reasons. Your eating pattern may be at an all time high when you were engaged in your aerobic activity. When you stop, it is still at an all time high; but you are not doing anything to burn off those extra calories. It is like going on a diet. When you get off your diet, your metabolism is sluggish, but you are eating more."

"But I eat the same amount as before."

"You may not realize that your calorie intake is above and beyond your daily requirement. It didn't happen overnight. Don't compare what you are eating from one day to the next, from one month to the next, or even from year to year if you were overeating during all that time.
Sure, you may find that there's no change in your eating habits if you were eating too much in the first place.
But if you compared the amount you are eating now to what you were eating *before you were doing your aerobic workout*, you may see a drastic difference."

"I don't know," you said rather dubiously. "As far back as I can remember, I always had the same portions and types of foods."

"The other possibility is that your diet could be high in fat. It's burned off when you are active; but once you stop exercising, it lingers around."

"That could be it," you said as you thought about it.

"Another possibility is that you do not have enough muscle mass to burn fat."

"Hmmm..." You also began to reflect on that.

"Those are separate topics by themselves which we will discuss later. The point I want to make here is that there is a difference between losing fat and striving for a set of 'washboard abs'. The latter suggests that your weight is more or less stable and that your waistline is already trimmed. But if you also want to take off those extra pounds of fat, then it is not just a matter of fine tuning your midsection; you also need an overhaul because even if you do manage to sculpt spectacular abs, their outline would not show through layers of fat.

That's why a lot of people give up when they do not see any definition. It may be there, but the problem is that it is hidden. If they were using a Device, they will probably discard it and complain that it is not functioning properly. But it may have been doing its job; it's just that they did not know about it.

Moreover, if a Device is primarily intended to produce rock hard abs, then losing weight will come painfully slow—if it's going to come at all. Sure, they may tell you on their infomercials that you will lose weight, but they will not say that it should be your *prime* concern. And the reason they do not come right out and say it is because their Devices are not intended primarily for losing weight.

It is important to realize at the outset that whenever I use the phrase 'losing weight', I actually mean 'slashing' that tire tube—or fat to be more specific."

"Why don't you say it then?" you declared impatiently.

"I use the term 'weight' for the benefit of those who are overweight. For them, the concept of weight and fat almost amount to the same thing. I want to let them know in a roundabout way—using terms that they understand—that my program also works for them.

But when it comes to losing it, the term *weight* and *fat* do not necessarily equal the same thing. There is the danger of losing much more than fat if you go about it the wrong way—like trying to lose it in a hurry by going on a crash diet.

That is the crux of the problem with some quick weight loss schemes. You cannot lose fat in a hurry—like in a matter of days—regardless of what the facts, figures, and endorsements tell you. The promoters will have you thinking the way they want you to think once you are caught with your guard, or pants, down—especially when you are at your flabbiest. You have to keep in mind that unlike carbohydrate, which is your body's primary fuel, fat burns slower. Sure, you may lose weight after several days if you resort to drastic measures like starving yourself, but you are not losing fat; most likely, you are losing something else which your body needs—like fluids or even muscles.

If you only have a slight bulge on your sides or front of your waist, it's possible for you to lose flab and maintain your weight—or you may even gain some weight—and still come out looking good. Fat is not as dense as muscle, so it is possible to get rid of excess fat and maintain your weight if you gain muscle at the same time. In fact, that is what will most likely happen if you start to eat right and exercise regularly."

5

The Intensity Factor

"OK, so what do I have to do?" you asked while feeling your sides—the main areas you wanted to "trim".

"It might surprise you that I do not advocate doing a hundred and one different types of exercises. In fact, I am just going to elaborate on a single exercise; the kind which the TV infomercials will tell you, 'It will not work.' You are just going to do sit-ups."

"What?" you declared with astonishment. "I was told that you can't burn fat with sit-ups. There's no such thing as 'spot reduction'. Fat comes off your body all at once. Besides—"

"Whoa! Hold on for a second," I tried to calm you down. "That is the general argument, but you also have to consider the mental as well as the physical context of my routine. The *intensity factor* involved when you do sit-ups my way will be just as or even more *intense* than an overall workout.

The usual notion of *intensity* is that you have to spend about half an hour or more doing a variety of exercises at a rate that will increase your pulse until you start to sweat.

But I have found that you can achieve an even higher degree of *intensity* around your midsection in a much shorter duration. The advantage of a high *intensity* and short duration program is that it reduces the tendency to quit due to boredom, self-discipline, or inconvenience."

"But I found that some workouts were pretty *intense*."

"That's true, but the main drawback is that the effect is not concentrated within the region where the fat mainly collects: around your abs."

"Why?"

"Let me answer that with an overview of my program. It provides a solution to the main excuses as to why some people do not do any exercises in the first place. Excuses like:
1. I do not have time.
2. I abhor exercises because I hate to get all sweaty and icky.
3. I do not like doing any sort of exercises in the first place.
4. I know that exercising is good for me: it jacks up my metabolic rate (and it can permanently set my metabolic rate higher if it is below average), burns calories, builds muscle which increases strength which in turn requires more fuel (fat being one of them) when it does work—but I am not motivated.
5. I tried exercising before, but I still cannot get my weight down."

"I hate to say this, but that just about sums up how I feel. But how would doing sit-ups make a difference?"

"Let's find out by providing some answers to those problems I mentioned:
My routine only takes 5 minutes a day—10 minutes if you are ambitious and if your schedule permits."

"And that's another thing—" you objected. You were starting to get excited again.

"I realize that fat takes longer to burn than carbohydrate," I acknowledged. "But sit-ups are the most *intense* form of exercise in terms of 'slashing your weight and trimming your abs'. You can increase this *physical intensity* by varying the way and the order that you do them. And you can boost it even further by means of the *multiplier effect*—a phenomenon which I came across while subjecting myself to various ways to lose weight. When you combine your *physical intensity* with the *multiplier effect*, you will end up with what I call the *intensity factor*.

It shortens the duration of your exercises, and that makes it comparatively easy to do them everyday. A full workout is not necessary. If you add the time you spend on your sit-ups in a month, it will probably come close to the time you spend on your overall workout during the same period. You are not engaged in your overall workout every day, but you are doing my shorter routine daily. Remember, if you miss a day at the gym, you lose an hour or so; but if you miss doing my sit-ups for a day, you lose only 5 to 10 minutes.

You will start off nice and slow, and you are not going to engage in anything strenuous. You should see results in about three months—even if you are still in phase one. If you only have a slight bulge, you will see results much quicker. That takes care of problem #1.

My exercises are not that difficult to do. It may 'feel' hard at the beginning if you did not do any sort of exercise for a long time. But there are different types of sit-ups with different levels of *intensity*, and you decide how fast you want to push yourself depending on how quickly your body adapts."

"It sounds compatible to what most people want from a home exercise program: to get the most out of it in the shortest time possible," you said from experience.

"Right. And empirical evidence from research in this area proves that 15 to 20 minutes of regular exercises can be just as beneficial as doing them over an extended period of time. But I have shortened the duration to only 5 to 10 minutes. Since you are not overexerting yourself, you will hardly work up a sweat. In fact, I used to go through my sets with my shirt and tie on before I head out to work. So that takes care of problem #2.

As for problem #3, don't think of sit-ups merely as an exercise. It is also a desensitizing drill when you do them the first thing in the morning and an hour before going to bed—the latter is optional, but it helps in the beginning when your struggling; it's like burning extra calories while you're sleeping.

By 'desensitizing', I mean you are slowly erasing the image of the person you hate to be and start replacing it with the sort of person you want to become. Visualizing this image of the new YOU is important, and I will explain why as we go along.

And my reply to problem #4 and #5 will brings us to the essence of my program: *You are reinforcing your mental commitment with your physical commitment and vice versa.*

Your will increase your chances of success when you apply two techniques that back each other up."

"Is this is another example of your tendency to offer 2 for 1's and no frills deals?"

"I suppose."

"Wouldn't it be better for business if you separate some of them and repackage each as a separate course?"

"Yeah, in some areas. But in others, you can't. It's all interconnected. That's what the *intensity factor* is all about. Besides, that's how you deal with a lack of motivation. I can go on and on talking to you until you *mentally* have the burning desire to do something, but it's not going to accomplish much until you *physically* do something. As with any exercise routine, begin doing it is half the battle."

"Tell me about it," you commented.

"A lot of people have difficult overcoming this hurdle—especially when it involves exercising every major muscle group in your body; you either do not have time for such a program, or you do not want to go to such extremes at first when all you want to do is to test the water. I try to remove this handicap by introducing only sit-ups; I will show you several variations, but all you need to do is to select four that you feel comfortable with. It can't get any simpler than that.

When you perform your first sit-up, you are actually kick starting the *process* involved in 'slashing your weight and trimming your abs'. It will work even if you refuse to do any other types of exercises in the future—although I hope it will stimulate you to try other kinds of activities to enhance your overall physique."

"You're kidding," you responded skeptically.

"Nope. And that's only the tip of the iceberg."

6

Sticking To It

"What you are also doing is that you are beginning to live the life of the person you want to become. One of the points I constantly emphasize is that once you begin to visualize the type of individual you really want to be, then you will be more incline to take the necessary steps to remove any obstacles that are preventing you from become that person.

To cut down on the time this would take due to daydreaming and/or just constantly talking about it instead of actually doing something, it would be a tremendous help if you actually took the first step—while you are visualizing the new YOU.

If you are serious about making a change, then you are actually saying, 'Yes, I intend to slash some weight and trim my abs.' Your *intention* is very important. It's the driving force behind getting what you want, and it also determines how long you can stick to that idea. The only piece of the picture that is missing is how you are going to initiate it. This is where your sit-ups come in.

And to make it easy for you, it's only 5 to 10 minutes in duration since a sit-up is a very *intense* form of exercise as far as 'slashing your weight and trimming your abs' goes."

"What about jogging or bicycling? Why aren't they intense?"

"They are—they benefit mainly your lower body. You will work up a good sweat, you may lose some weight, your legs may acquire great definition; I recommend it. But I am talking about bottling that *intensity* and applying it to a more specific region. I have a lot of joggers in my class whose abs are not that well defined. Of course, jogging helps; but there is still a lot of room for improvement. The *intensity* from such a workout is still disperse as far as 'slashing your weight and trimming your abs' goes. What I want to do is to confine your efforts to an area where most of your fat collects."

"Around my abs?"

"That's right. Moreover, you can make use of that *intensity* to adopt the *proper intention*. Getting started and having a game plan is one thing, but it is also important to continue doing it.

If you had tried certain exercises and gave up, it's because you were not applying the *proper intensity*, both mentally and physically, to achieve the kind of changes you want. Starting out with the wrong *intensity* is one of the main reasons why a lot of gut-busting equipments are lying dormant and collecting dust in basements across the country. The owners may have felt very enthusiastic at first when they tried them out, but their interest gradually dwindled because of a mismatch between what they desired and what those gadgets could actually offer.

You need to have the *proper intensity* before you can maintain the *proper intention*. Of course, you may have the *proper intention* and visualization even if your routine does not quite deliver the *proper intensity*; but at some point in time, the lack of the *proper intensity* will catch up to you. You will just give up when your expectations are not met.

Once you have the *proper intensity*, it will induce the same *intensity* in your *intention* to lose weight—something that's often termed as 'sheer determination'. Some people have it to start with, but a lot of people who want to lose weight don't. That's why I suggest you start developing it. Even if you think you are determined enough, it doesn't hurt to reinforce it."

"In other words, the *proper intensity* will give me the strength to *stick* to my commitment and to do what it takes to become the new ME," you posited.

"Exactly. You are actually strengthening your mind as well as your body. Once they are synchronized, it's quite a motivational booster because you will see results in the short term. If you see a string of improvements within a few months, it will definitely help you to press on.

It's a waste of time doing sit-ups just for the sake of doing them. It's not just a matter of going through the motions. You also have to remind yourself why you are doing them—namely, your mission statement or affirmation: *'Yes, I intend to slash some weight and trim my abs.'*

Once that is clearly etched in your mind along with the image of the new YOU, you are actually striving to perform a host of other things that a lean healthy person would do. In fact, you are engaging yourself in that sort of life style, or as you put it: *sticking* to your commitment.

At the conscious level, this means that you are reinforcing your will power and gradually becoming more selective in what you eat, avoiding foods that are dripping with fat, increasing your carbohydrate intake, cutting down or eliminating your snacking, continuing to do your exercises, exploring other avenues to boost your cardiovascular and strength, et cetera.

Once the sit-ups stimulate your *intention* to 'slash your weight and trim your abs' at the conscious level, your *intention* and your visualization will gradually be embedded deeper and deeper as you progress. At some point your *intention* will change into *determination*.

The more determine you become, the more liable your thoughts will affect your mental processes at the subconscious level. And that, in turn, will reprogram the internal functions of your body. When you are thinking 'lean' with enough *determination* and with the proper mental image, you are giving your subconscious mind a new set of information. To achieve this 'lean' look, it will regulate your craving for food, maintain your proper metabolism, correct inconsistent biochemical reactions, stabilize the function of various organs, et cetera—just when you think that those things were beyond your control."

"Hmmm... So it all starts with the physical process of doing sit-ups."

"That's your *physical commitment*," I pointed out.

"And then the visualization of the new ME along with my affirmation comes next."

"And that's your *mental commitment*."

"That's all I have to do?"

"That's it...for now."

7

The Catalyst

"Couldn't I just employ visualization and forget about the sit-ups?"

"It's an interesting idea. Visualization is a technique that some people adopt when they want to accomplish a difficult task. By picturing the outcome often enough beforehand, they hope that it will unfold accordingly. But when it comes to losing a few pounds, there is another condition you have to satisfy: you also have to be physically engaged in the act of 'slashing' your weight. That will become obvious if you attempt to wish yourself thin by being inactive—by just sitting in front of the TV for instance.

We all tend to procrastinate. If it is hard to commit ourselves to 'slash' our weight, then the additional task of 'trimming' our abs will be a very tall order. To overcome this hurdle, I have made the actual means of taking the first step as simple and as *effective* as possible: by doing a single exercise for a minimum of only 5 minutes.

The key word is *effective*. If it is simple but not *effective*, it is not going to work. I have already mentioned that sit-ups by themselves are *intense*. This is nothing mysterious. There are certain activities which are more *intense* than others—like shovelling snow for example; but sit-ups do not have any of its adverse features, and that's another benefit that makes it *effective*. According to the Journal of The American Medical Association, shovelling snow puts more strain on the heart than a heavy exercise session. After you do it for two minutes, your heart rate will exceed the upper limit commonly found after an aerobic workout. Although doing sit-ups do not restrict the flow of blood as severely as shovelling snow—and thus making your heart work harder—get a medical check up before you start exercising.

You can make a sit-up even more *intense* by isolating your efforts to a smaller area—without restricting an adequate flow of blood. This is where your ability to focus plays a big part. When you do your sit-ups, concentrate on the part of your abs that you want to improve. For example, if you are doing your regular 'crunches', concentrate on the upper abs since a front 'crunch' targets that area. When you are doing your reverse 'crunch', concentrate on your lower abs. When you are doing your side sit-ups, concentrate on your obliques or side abs.

Sometimes all you need to do is to make a minor adjustment to get the most out of your workout. If you are doing you side sit-ups, for instance, it makes a big difference if you turn a little more to one side, if you lean slightly farther back, or if you slow down your movement. By practising you concentration, you will eventually feel what adjustment should be made to further isolate a specific group of muscle to handle the work. It's like shifting around in a new chair to find which position is best.

But your comfort index will change as you continue to make progress. What was uncomfortable a month ago will become tolerable. When you workout, always try to go a bit outside your comfort zone."

"Wouldn't that be painful?"

"I'm glad you bought that up. Pain is something I want to talk more about in a few minutes. For now, just remember that any adjustment that produces more work will take more effort, and that is what you should be striving for.

It will be less painful if you relax. Relaxation helps to improve blood circulation, and that will provide more oxygen to your muscles. Since fat needs oxygen to burn, it's also a good idea to teach your body to maintain that relaxation after your workout."

"How do you do that?"

"When you flex and unflex your ab muscles as you sit-up and lean back, tell yourself to relax throughout the movement and not just when you unflex."

"What if someone is not relaxed in the first place?"

"When you lie on the floor or on a bench to do your sit-ups, close your eyes and tell yourself to relax before you start your routine. Repeat the key word, 'relax', to yourself a few times. You have to retrain specific groups of muscles to relax. Start by stretching your facial muscles with a smile; then let go and allow your jaw to drop. Do not clench your teeth. Then tell the muscles around your neck, shoulders, arms, chest, stomach, and legs to relax by tightening each of them and letting go.
Go over the process again if you still feel tense. Later, you will be able to become totally relaxed with a single command instead of performing a series of mental massages.
You will find that your routine will become easier even though you are expending the same amount energy."

"And this will make my sit-ups more *effective*?"

"Yes, and from here, you can actually take it to another *intensity* level."

"You're kidding."

"Nope. That's why it is important to have the proper mental image. It acts as a catalyst."

"You just mentioned that visualization will help me stick to my commitment. Are you also saying that it will boost the outcome of my sit-ups?"

"That's right. The *proper* mental image of the new YOU acts as a *multiplier*. It helps to bring about a phenomenon which I call the *multiplier effect* which I will explain in more detail in a minute. But it can only happen if you have the *proper visualization*. If the image is there one day and not the next or if it is fuzzy, then the *multiplier effect* will give you a different set of results.

You must start with the *proper physical intensity* to deepen the impression of your visualization and your *intention*.

That will produce the *proper mental commitment* at the conscious and subconscious level. Once you get this far, your mind will regulate your body in the manner I just described.

What this will actually do is that it will makes your body more receptive to your sit-ups. This is where the *multiplier effect* comes in to boost the *physical intensity* of your sit-ups.

The usual notion is that only the *physical intensity* is involved when you perform your exercises. The *mental intensity* is often ignored. And that is too bad because it's the *mental intensity* (which is actually the *intensity* of your *visualization* and your *intention*) that often makes a difference. Once it brings the *multiplier effect* into play, it can boost your *physical intensity* dramatically."

"Suppose I don't do the sit-ups. Will the *multiplier* boost whatever other activity I'm engaged in?"

"Even if it does, those 'other activities' may not be as *intense* as a sit-up, and it may not focus that *intensity* directly on your abs."

"And the flip side is that if I don't employ visualization, I will just be depending on my sit-ups," you began to realize.

"By removing the catalyst, you will just be relying on the physical aspect of the *intensity factor*. I'm not saying that sit-ups by themselves will not work. It might take a longer time if you are not as determined as you should be.

Besides, it is also a confidence booster. When you do your sit-ups and visualize the outcome before you go to work, for example, you feel good about yourself. It is like putting on your best clothes."

"Is that how you visualize yourself?"

"Sure. I feel more comfortable and confident in certain situations when I know that I am putting my best foot forward. When I perform my sit-ups, it is like slipping on an invisible girdle. I can feel that it improves whatever outer garment I have on."

"How long will it take before I can feel good about myself in this way?"

"Immediately. Visualize it. You are picturing yourself as how others see you."

"Am I missing something here?" you questioned. You were a bit puzzled. "Is this different from visualizing how I want to look?"

"Not really." I want to clarify. "It's all part of the new YOU. Some people tend to forget how *they* want to look; they worry more about how other people see them and pay less attention to how they see themselves. When that happens, they will often end up with a distorted image, and that can lead to all sorts of problems.

If you worry too much about how people see you, then you might take extreme measures—like going on a crash diet and lose more weight than you have to just to please others. The worse part is that you might even do this subconsciously.

You have to realize that the shape you want to be in is compatible with the views of the majority of the people you meet everyday. You control how others see you as well as how you see yourself."

"How could I physically control—" you interrupted.

"It all takes place mentally. If you distort that image, it's your mind that is playing tricks on you. It's a hallucination. No one did it to you, you did it to yourself. Only you can undo it by making the proper mental adjustment and start visualizing properly."

"But not everyone will see me as how I would see myself," you argued.

"If you visualize yourself as healthy and fit, 99.9% of the people you meet will agree with that picture if they can see the image you see. The other .1% is not worth considering. Otherwise, you will end up trying to please everyone.

Then the process will be painfully slow since you know very well that in real life you cannot please everyone; your vision of your true self will keep shifting."

"What about the real me? It's a reminder that I'm not cut exactly like the way I want to see myself?"

"But we are just talking about visualization. The image of the person that you are striving to become is the issue here. Besides, who is the real YOU? The person that you see in the mirror before you right now can always be improved. So how do you want to improve yourself? According to the whims and fancies of a fickle few? According to doubts and uncertainties? Or according to the real YOU?

Remember, the image that you have of yourself is like a catalyst or *multiplier*. If you distort the image of the real YOU, then you will take steps to make that distorted image a reality, consciously and subconsciously," I emphasized.

8

The Multiplier Effect

"The sequence of events in the total process goes something like this:

Do your sit-ups. State your mission statement or affirmation. Visualize its outcome with the image of the new YOU. Your visualization acts as a medium and as a catalyst. It transmits your intention to your conscious and subconscious mind and stimulates them to comply with your instructions. It acts as a multiplier in the sense that your body will eventually become more receptive to the effect of your sit-ups."

"So you're saying that it's possible to see results in a shorter time?"

"Sure. That's why I call it this mental portion of the *intensity factor* the *multiplier effect*. It contributes a lot to your overall effort; remember, when you reinforce the image of the new YOU with your sit-ups, it affects not just your conscious mind—the subconscious is also activated.

Your subconscious mind does two things: It stimulates your body to identify with the new YOU. Then it makes your body more responsive to exercises; this is where your sit-ups come in during phase one along with any other types of exercises you might be interested in during phase two.

When you think about it, you are actually exercising your mind as well as your abs when you do your sit-ups.

The kids in my martial arts class go through the same sort of training to overcome their fears. They reinforce the image of how they will react in a real situation by doing the actual drills over and over again. Later, I will check their progress by setting up various situations to simulate conditions on the streets.

You can easily test your own progress by observing your reaction to junk food. For example, do you control yourself or do you nibble and snack incessantly?"

"You ever try waving a triple layered chocolate cake in front of those in your weight loss class?" you wondered.

"It's an interesting suggestion," I said while making a mental note. "But they have just started. Maybe I can try it later."

"You would actually conduct such a test?" you asked. You didn't expected me to take you seriously.

"Sure. Why not? They have to be conditioned mentally as well as physically. If they have a sweet tooth or if they snack incessantly, the mental image of the shape they want to be in will have to be reinforced. They can do that by modifying their affirmation, and I will tell you how to do that in a moment—or they can motivate themselves with the progress they make in the short term, and that's what they are trying to do now. In fact, I think they will see some positive results very shortly since they are also doing other types of exercises besides sit-ups."

"I though you said it was not necessary to do other types of exercises," you reminded me.

"You don't have to during phase one—or even phase two, but it does help.

Engaging in an overall workout without paying enough attention to your abs will not be much help. But an overall workout plus 5 to 10 minutes of abdominal work will do more for your *overall* physique than what an abdominal routine alone can do.

It all depends on what *you* want. A rippling upper and lower body as well as rock hard abs? A toned upper and lower body as well as rock hard abs? A somewhat rippling and partial toned upper and lower body plus a set of rock hard abs? More of one and less of another? Or do you just want to 'slash your weight and trim your abs'?

It also depends on how much time you want to give up, your commitment, and your determination."

"I don't know…" you said hesitantly.

"That's why I suggest you wait until phase two before you decide on how you want to supplement your sit-ups. By then you will have a better perspective of what you want, and your determination will be more intact."

"Will the *multiplier effect* target my abs if I was only engaged in an overall workout?"

"That's a good question. The affirmation I suggested you to repeat when you do your routine—and even when you are not doing them—will contribute more to your *intention* of 'slashing your weight and trimming your abs' than to an affirmation that pertains to an overall workout."

"You mean it depends on what a person's *intention* is when he or she decides to do an overall workout?"

"That's right. In the majority of cases, an overall mission statement is not specific enough. It does not pinpointing the fat burning process to a particular region. A lot of experts, however, would say that this cannot be done—that the burning of fuel takes place throughout your body."

"That seems to be the common consensus."

"Well, tell me then, if you *intend* to trim fat from your midsection, would you rather be doing push-ups, squats, bench presses, lateral raises, curls, et cetera?"

You thought about it for awhile and then shrugged your shoulders.

"You will get good definition in your arms, shoulders, chest, and legs; but what about your abs?

I have students in my martial arts class who are very fit. Their fitness consciousness are at the level where they would work out for an hour or so before coming to my class. In fact, they work out about three times a week. They have great definition in their arms, shoulders, chest, lats, thighs, calves—but there is this one section that sticks out like a sore thumb. You guessed it—their abs.

I am not denying that fuel is burnt throughout your body, but I think you can still make it burn more *intense* in your midsection by doing sit-ups within the proper mental and physical context."

"Weren't they doing any ab work?"

"Yes they were, but their *intention* was different. They were relaying a different message to their conscious and subconscious mind, so the outcome was different."

"Didn't they have the proper visualization?"

"Sure, but then again, their *intention* was different."

"What's the difference between the two?"

"Before your mental image can act as a catalyst, the *proper* ingredients must be present. You need to have the *proper intention* along with the *proper mission statement* or *affirmation*.

Your affirmation is a verbal expression of your *intention*, and it is also an interpretation of what you are visualizing. That's what I meant when I said that the image you have of yourself acts as a medium and as a catalyst. It acts as a medium when it transmits your affirmation to your conscious and subconscious mind. It acts as a catalyst when that image is steady, focused, and embedded deep in your thoughts.

If you take away one of those ingredients, it may not mold your body exactly to the shape you desire."

"You mean my visualization by itself is not enough?"

"If I just visualize myself as an ox without affirming that I want to be as strong as an ox, it doesn't mean I will turn into an ox. That's not spelled out in my affirmation. In fact, nothing was spelled out, so nothing will happen.

But even if I did spell it out—that I want to be as strong as an ox—it doesn't mean I will receive a set of washboard abs. The statement is too general, and I may end up with a massive upper and lower body while my waistline remained unchanged—since I didn't say anything about 'slashing my weight'.

You have to be specific in your set of instructions on how to assemble what you are visualizing. That's where your *intention* and *affirmation* come in.

When you visualize the new YOU while repeating to yourself that you want to lose weight, then that's what you will get if the image of the new YOU corresponds with your affirmation. If you also put in a request for a set of trimmed abs, you will get that too if the mental image matches your affirmation."

"Can I list as many requests as I want?"

"It depends on your commitment. How bad do you want it? What steps are you willing to take to get it?"

"There's always a catch," you muttered.

"But sometimes it's worth the extra effort."

9

Getting Physical

But there was something about this *intensity factor*—the mental side of it was OK, you can live with that, no sweat. But as far as the physical side was concerned, you still suspected that there might be a lot of work involved despite the fact that I said it would only take 5 to 10 minutes a day. Images of performing lots and lots of sit-ups flashed across your mind, and you began to calculate how many you could actually do within that period. The number that you came up with paled in comparison to what you thought was ideal.

"Isn't there a better way?"

"Like what?"

"Couldn't I start with the latest state-of-the-art gadget for my abs instead?"

"You could, but you are taking a risk. It may not give what you want in a short time. You can expect to relapse back to your old self if you do not see any short term results. In fact, some of them do not work even in the long term. It's like saying, 'OK, I'm ready to write the Great North American Novel.' You may actually sit down and do it. But when you find that you are not getting anywhere after a month, you will likely give up on the project.

Little did you realize that tackling the Great North American Novel, like losing weight, may take longer than you anticipated. If you do not see any short term gains in the process or if you are not aware of them, you are going to forget about the whole idea—unless you are that rare individual who can bear all pain and disappointment regardless of what happens."

"Why can't I get any short term results?" you asked.

"There are several reasons, and I will go over each of them in turn. But the main one is that the *intensity factor* is missing if you rely strictly on your Device."

"Couldn't I tie that in to a Device somehow."

"It depends. A lot of Devices lack the proper *intensity*—that is, the *physical intensity* component of the *intensity factor*. If you're off to a bad start, you may not be spending 5 to 10 minutes as we originally planned; and that in turn will throw your short term expectations off schedule—not to mention the dampening effect that this will have on your mental commitment.
When you do a sit-up without the constraints found in some Devices that restrict your movement or position, you can increase your *load* much more. I mean, try doing 10 'crunches' on an ab bench set at the steepest angle and tell me whether or not you feel it.
Although some Devices have different *physical intensity* levels, they are either limited, or the shift from one level to the next poses too much of a load for the average person; and that is why a lot of people are stuck at the first level—and thus retarding any progress.
The most *intense* form of sit-ups, by the way, is when you try to do your 'crunches' while you are dangling upside down. It's one of the ways I make use of one of the Pilates equipment: 'The Rack'," I pointed out on your pamphlet.

"Ouch," you cringed. "That looks stressful."

1

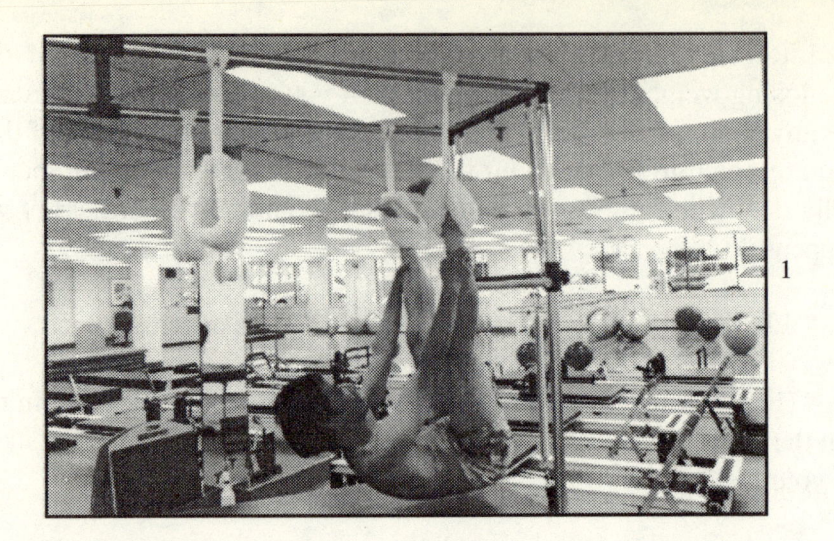

"Only when you try to place a load on yourself too soon or when you try to overdo it—beyond the number of repetitions that you are comfortable with. That's the point I want to make here."

"Well, there is this one gut-buster Device I tried, and I found that I could go on and on and on," you recalled.

"If you can do 50 sit-ups on that Device and only 10 of them the old fashion way (on the ab bench or otherwise), then that tells me you are expending more *work* the old fashion way. And it also tells me that your abs are not as developed as they should be.

The amount of work you do plays an important part in determining the *physical intensity* in the kinds of exercises that you are doing, and that in turn contributes to the outcome of your efforts.

Work is the expenditure of energy when you perform your sit ups. There are two ways you can increase the work you do:

1. By increasing the number or repetition. Performing 100 sit-ups, for example, takes more effort than doing 10 sit-ups.

2. By increasing the load. Performing 100 sit-ups with a load of 50 pounds on your chest, for instance, takes more effort than doing them without such a load. The heavier the load you place on your abs, the harder it is for you to do your sit-ups; and that means you have to do more work.

If you do a lot of hard work by increasing the repetition or load, you expend a lot of energy in the form of heat. You will burn more calories; that in turn, plays an important part in determining how much fat is being trimmed. Of course, carbohydrate is also burned along with fat. To ensure that you are not just burning carbohydrate, the length of your exercises—that involve only sit-ups—should be at least 5 minutes."

"That's within a mental as well as physical context," you broke in.

"That's correct. A lot of Devices fail because there is the absence of the proper *physical intensity* to start with. Even when the *multiplier effect* kicks in, there is still a lot of room for improvement.

If a Device allows you to do work relatively easy, then you are not applying the proper load, and you are not doing enough work. You can make up for that by increasing the number of repetitions. But after you get used to doing that, it can get pretty boring if you end up doing a lot of sit-ups—not to mention a waste of time if your abs do not look or feel any different.

That's the trouble with some rocking-back-and-forth type of Devices. Your lats—the muscles running along your sides and back—actually help you lift yourself up. Your abs are getting some workout, but you would benefit more from the old fashion way of doing sit-ups since your abs will be doing most of the work. Another drawback with such Devices is that it is hard for your obliques to be properly strengthen by rocking back and forth. Even if you expose them to a load, it may not be enough since the range of movement is restricted, and your upper body (and sometimes even your lower body) is supported by a headrest instead of allowing its total weight to bear down on your abs.

There are other Devices that allow you to adjust the load. But is it totally directed against your abs or does your arms and/or other parts of your body participate to take up most of it? This is one of the problems with a lot of the pushing and pulling type of gadgets; you are likely to exercise your biceps more. But do you want big biceps or well define abs?

Some Devices benefit your biceps, triceps, shoulders, lats, back, quads, and hamstrings as well as your abs."

"But some do allow you to change the *intensity*."

"Like I said, sometimes each incremental increase is too much of a jump. It is not dictated by your comfort level. That means you will progress a lot slower. In some instances, you will not progress at all if the initial load becomes very easy to do after awhile. It's possible to be stuck doing a lot of easy repetition without gaining enough strength to manage the load at the next level.

It's like doing 'curls' with a 5 pound dumbbell when you know you can perform the same number of 'reps' with 20 pounds. You are limiting the development of your muscles if the displacement requires almost no effort."

"But aren't there others that isolate the efforts against your abs?"

"Sure, but sometimes you can get the same sort of feeling by doing isometrics—by just tightening up your abs. In some cases, you really have to tighten them up to prevent injury because some Devices make you 'feel' it in more ways than one—especially when they have protruding parts that stab right into your midsection. So even though you 'feel' it, the proper load is missing.

There are claims that some Devices can firm up your midsection in half the time as sit ups by concentrating the work on your abs. But if you modify the way you do your sit-ups, you will find that your efforts will be even more concentrated.

You can't just pick any sort of exercise haphazardly if you want to 'slash your weight and trim your abs'. The sit-ups that I have chosen are for specific parts of your abs, and that extra isolation makes them even more *intense*. The front 'crunch' targets your upper abs, the reverse 'crunch' targets your lower abs, and the side sit-up targets your left and right obliques.

To turn the *physical intensity* level up another notch, you must:

1. Gradually increase the number of repetitions. If you can just do 10 sit-ups on your first day, that is OK—as long you intend to increase that amount.

2. Have the proper load—not just directed *at* your abs, but *only* for your abs. In other words, your abs should do most of the work.

I suggest that you keep increasing your 'reps' first until you hit your target: like a total of 100 sit-ups a day for example."

"Is that how many I should be doing?" you asked.

"No. That is only an arbitrary number. Some people can do much more, but you will probably do less than that if you have not done any sort of workout for a long time. I am not saying that your repetitions should be effortless. On the other hand, I do not believe that you have to push yourself until you are rolling in pain. A 'no pain no gain' attitude can easily dampen your motivation.

What I do suggest is that your repetition should be just within your threshold of pain—not excruciating pain; rather, it's a sort of pain which you can take."

"How much pain?" you asked a little nervous.

"It's a mild pain that produces a slightly burning sensation in your body. It is a sign that you are burning fuel. You may not achieve it at first, but the number of sit-ups needed to produce this condition is what you should be striving for. A lot of people are not aware that this type of mild pain usually accompanies this plateau. In fact, it's not actually pain—but a 'tightness' that is often misinterpreted as pain."

"How can you tell the difference?" you wanted to clarify.

"If you feel excruciating pain, you muscles seize up and you cannot continue; but if you do your sit-ups right, there would be plenty of warning ahead of time before you would end up like that. There would be several stages of 'tightness' you have to go through first, and it becomes less and less tolerable as you come closer to real pain. So if you feel 'tight' during the first stage, it is still possible to go on until you reach the second stage; and that is when I usually stop to take a breather.

When you reached the first stage of 'tightness', try to maintain it as long as possible. It is not unusual to do another 5 or 10 more sit-ups. Some people can prolong this sensation to enable the burning of fat to peak by doing as much as 40 to 50 more. This is not necessary, but it's nice if you can do it—and you can, with practise.

After a month or two, you will find that the 'tightness' will be less pronounced. How many repetitions you should do before you become engaged in the next level of pain (mild pain, that is) depends on your age, health, biological make-up, et cetera. However, do your exercises gradually at the beginning, and do not push yourself more than necessary.

Again, it is not necessary to torture yourself until you are crumbling in agony; nor is it necessary to be dripping in sweat before you see any results. In fact, you may not produce any sweat at all since you are just exercising your abs."

"How can you burn fat without sweating?" you asked. You seemed a little confused.

"It all has to do with the *intensity factor*. When you do your sit-ups for the first time, this burning sensation may not feel *intense*. But once you start doing more, you will feel the difference. When you get to the point where you can achieve your initial target with ease, then you may have to increase your repetition.

Keep doing that at different intervals until you feel that you are spending more time than necessary to finish your workout. For example, if you can only spare 5 minutes in the morning, and it is taking you 10 minutes, then you may have to increase the load instead of going on and on without noticing any difference. Once you increase the load, the number of repetitions may drop; that is OK if you still feel that those calories are being converted to heat. And you will not be dripping in sweat if you only intend to exercise for 5 minutes."

"Then you start building your 'reps' back up again?"

"Yes, but before you do that, make sure that you have established the *proper* load. You can do hundreds of sit-ups everyday, but it will have little effect if it is not followed by a certain degree of 'tightness'. It's like bending your arms up and down hundreds of times each day for a month. Are your biceps getting any bigger? No, because you have not applied the *proper* load. Repeat the process with the *proper* weights, and you will see some results.

Everybody has a different *physical intensity* level. If the sit-ups are not producing the results that you want, then you have to make an adjustment. It is useless to keep doing something that does not work.

If you are very fit, for example, and you just want to do something about your spongy midsection, then most likely you will have to increase your load once you get used to your sit-ups.

You have the capacity to do harder work; and if you don't put in the required effort, you will not coax your muscles to get larger—and that is the only way your abs will ripple. It may mean engaging in the more difficult variety of sit-ups, doing them on an ab bench, applying an external load, experiment with them in different orders, doing them in sets, or employing a combination of such techniques—which I will explain in a moment.

But if you are somewhat out of shape, then you may take a different approach—like adjusting your position to ease the load in order to gradually get used to it, scheduling your workout at an optimum time, doing double time by doing your sit-ups an hour or so before you go to bed as well as during the morning, et cetera. You have to be a bit creative to see what works best for you."

"Building muscles is one thing, but what about losing weight?"

"Don't forget it's all part of the *intensity factor*. It's a 2 in 1 approach, remember?

Like I said before, you do not have to 'tone' your body one day by engaging in activities like jogging and swimming and building 'body mass' the next by pumping weights.

When you increase the load, you are increasing the *physical intensity*. And when you increase the *physical intensity*, you are increasing the *multiplier effect*. And when you increase the *multiplier effect*, you increase your capacity to lose weight as well as to build body mass.

Your muscles will also help you burn fat. That's one of the main reasons why a bodybuilder's weight is stable. But you don't have to worry about excessively huge muscles. Your ab muscles can only get so big. It doesn't bulge like your major muscles in your arms and legs.

Although this *process* of 'toning' and building strength will take place at the same time, you will slim down first before you will notice any definition.

Another thing to keep in mind is that your *intention* and visualization will also trigger you to make a conscious and subconscious effort to lose weight. You will be more selective in what you eat. You will avoid foods that goes against the grain of achieving the new YOU."

"It all starts with doing sit-ups," you began to ponder that thought again.

"Your *physical intensity* level will change. It will be low in the beginning, and you will adopt a higher level as you progress; and don't forget, at some point it will level off. It makes more sense to ease into it rather than going gung ho on the first day.

In my case, I just do a total of 150 sit-ups on the ab bench which include side sit-ups and front and reverse 'crunches'. I don't have to do 200 plus. But it does not mean I would never do it. Maybe I'll take a stab at it one or two days in a month when I'm in the mood, but it's not necessary to do it everyday. Doing my 'reps' in the range of 150 or so works for me because that's the number I feel comfortable with—after establishing the *proper* load."

"About 150 or so," you began to repeat to yourself. It was not as bad as you thought. But still...

"That was after I got used to doing them. When you start, you may do a lot less. But as long as you intend to boost your number of 'reps' as you go along, it's no problem.

A word of caution: if you increased the load by resorting to external weights, by carrying a dumbbell for example, make sure that it is not excessive. And do not increase the load that often. Your lower back can only take so much.

Also, don't forget about what I said about how your *mental attitude* fits into all this. I am not saying that sit-ups by themselves will not work. Having the proper repetition and load are the keys to seeing quick short term results. With the proper mental commitment, you can speed it up even more."

"Hmmm…" you replied with a nod. "I wonder if this will work for my cousin Jane."

"You sound like she has given up hope."

"She has—since nothing seems to work for her."

"Well, let me tell you a story about someone who also had a lot of trouble losing weight…"

10

A Prime Example

"To reiterate, your main concern at first is to shed fat and trim your abs. You may even end up with a set of washboard abs as a bonus during phase one if you are not excessively overweight. You are going to accomplish that with one exercise: sit-ups."

"You sound like those promoters on TV," you commented.

"Sure, each of them thinks that his or her program is the best in the world. I do not know how my ranks, but it does have the following differences:
 1. I have tested it on myself.
 2. I offered it to selected students in my martial arts class.
 3. It's been adopted by people who have difficulty losing weight—people like Mr. Michael Faulkner who used to struggle with his weight problem for over 20 years. You can see his results for yourself. Compare the 'before' picture in figure 2 to his 'after' picture in figure 3 in your workbook," I pointed out.

"He did this just by doing sit-ups?" you questioned somewhat in disbelief.

"He's the living proof that doing sit-ups the old fashion way can work wonders for your abs—not to mention your weight."

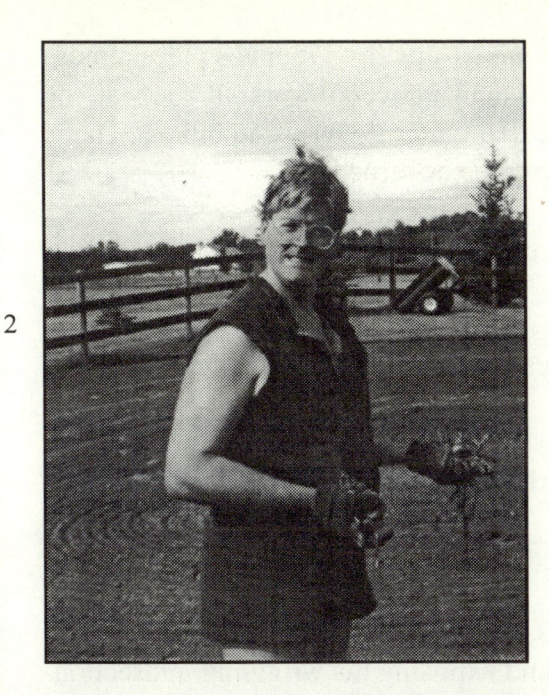

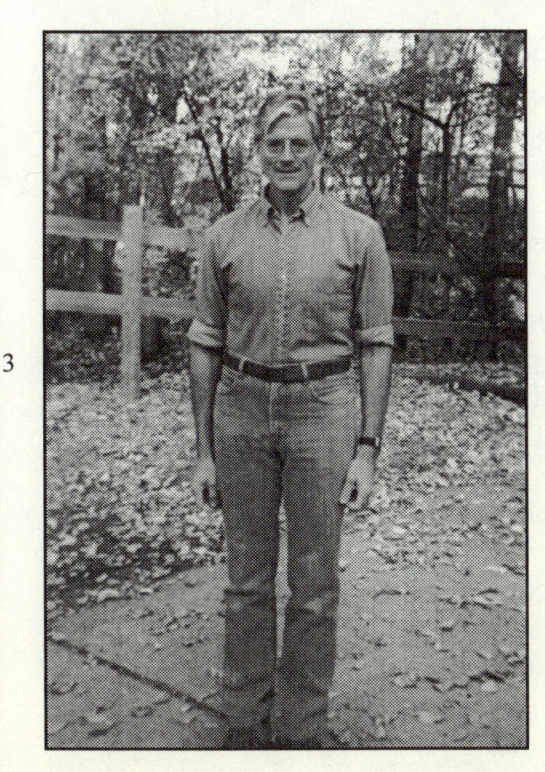

"My cousin Jane would love to meet him."

"That could be arranged."

"But it still seems to go against the conventional wisdom which flatly states that you need to do a total workout—without any ands, ifs, or buts about it," you brought that argument up again.

"That may be so if you want to strengthen all your major muscle groups. But you are just interested in a specific section: your abs. Besides, I have seen people who go to the gym 5 days a week for a year pumping iron to the point of injuring their wrists and elbow joints—not to mention the hidden injuries to the disks of their spines and knees and to their hip cartilages. You can see bulk throughout their bodies as a result of the tremendous load they subjected themselves to; but again, the only type of bulk that remains unchanged is in their midsection.

They have the right idea that the *intensity factor* should come into play. But why not apply it to the area where most of the fat is collected?

Your *intensity factor* from doing sit-ups for 5 minutes plays a more effective role in sculpting your abs than an overall workout. I repeat, the magic number is 5 minutes a day, 10 minutes if you are ambitious. That's all you need to do as far as sit-ups are concerned."

"Does it really work?" you inquired while continuing to compare both illustrations.

"Sure. Ask Michael. He represents those who find it very difficult to lose weight."

"My cousin have the same problem."

"Then they have something in common. Let me tell you about Michael's story.
When he was 18, he was 240 pounds. His worst fear was taking his shirt off at his high school gym and exposing his wriggling midsection. "Oh my God, don't let me be a 'skin'," he used to say whenever teams had to be selected.
Twenty-six years later, he decided that enough is enough; it all started when he went to Sears for a new suit and found that a size 44 no longer fits. He needed a 46. He used the memory from that incident as fuel to get off the couch and do something—like getting rid of a few pounds.
He knew that it would take some work because it was the second time that he was overweight. His weight between the ages of 36 to 44 was the mirror image of what he was like when he was from 9 to 20.
He started smoking and dieting when he was 20, and that seems to work for awhile. He lost a 100 pounds. He remembered that moment vividly when he weighed himself on a scale in Sydney, Australia where he used to live back in July of 1972. He was 22 then."

"You can lose weight by smoking?"

"It's possible. Nicotine can reduce your desire to eat by affecting the activity of serotonin and dopamine which are substances that control your appetite; nicotine also causes your adrenal glands to release catecholamines which in turn cause the liver to release glucose into the bloodstream and your fat cells to release fatty acids. Your body receives more energy, and your appetite is reduced. That is the good news. The bad news is that you have to maintain the habit.

Once you quit, that's another story. Even if you do not consume more calories, there is still the tendency to gain weight. As a result of biochemical changes when you quit smoking, your body's tendency to store fat may go up as a result of a decrease in your metabolic rate. What's more scary is that a portion of your carbohydrate intake can now end up as fat as a result of an increase in insulin activity. In other words, when the insulin level in your blood goes up, it is easier for glucose to be transported into your muscles. Excess glucose is converted to fat. And to make things worst, your appetite may increase—especially for sweets.

And that's what happened to Michael.

When he quit smoking in 1986, he weighted 150 pounds. He expected to gain back around 15 pounds; instead, he gained back 86 pounds over the next 8 years. When he weighted in at 236 pounds on January of 1994, he made a daring decision to get his weight down to 200 pounds by March 1994. But when the moment of truth arrived, he had surpassed his goal; he had trimmed down to an amazing 196 pounds."

"How did he do it?" You sounded less skeptical and became more interested in the actual process.

"Simple. By concentrating on one exercise: sit-ups. He would just hook his foot under a solid support and away he went. During that period he did an average of 200 sit-ups a day, and the most he did was around 400.

But he did one other thing during those months: he refrained from snacking—something which was almost as hard as exercising. 'But the old cliche that your body is a temple began to make sense the more weight I lost,' he told me. 'Once I started losing weight, however, I would still treat myself to a snack. I do not drink alcohol—hardly at all.'

When he started, he could only do 25 sit-ups, and the next day his abs 'hurt like hell'. He had to cut it down to 5, but he did not give up. In fact, he became obsessive. When the pain subsided, he began doing 5 more; then 10 more a few days after that, then 15 more, 20 more—then it became multiples of 10's and 20's.

It got to the point where on a good day he could do 1600 sit ups. 'But I could actually go on and on all day. If I do stop at 1600, it would be due to boredom or time constraint rather than anything else.'

To save time and to make it more challenging, he added 80 pound weight plates on his chest. 'Actually it's not that hard,' he said modestly. 'Most of my height is from my legs. So the mechanics of doing sit-ups is to my advantage.'

Figure 4 in your workbook shows Michael's way of increased the 'load' once his number of repetitions fell into the four digit category," I pointed out.

"That's very impressive. How long do you think it would take for me to get back in shape?"

"You are not *that* out of shape."

"The main problem are these bulges on my sides," you said as you grabbed a handful.

"Those 'handles', as they're sometimes called, are typical—even on someone who constantly works out. A lot of people believe that it's impossible to get rid of them, but it's not. I have designed my side-sit ups to target them. But you also have to do your front and reverse 'crunches' too to take up the slack. Again, it only takes 5 minutes a day—10 minutes if you really want to get going.

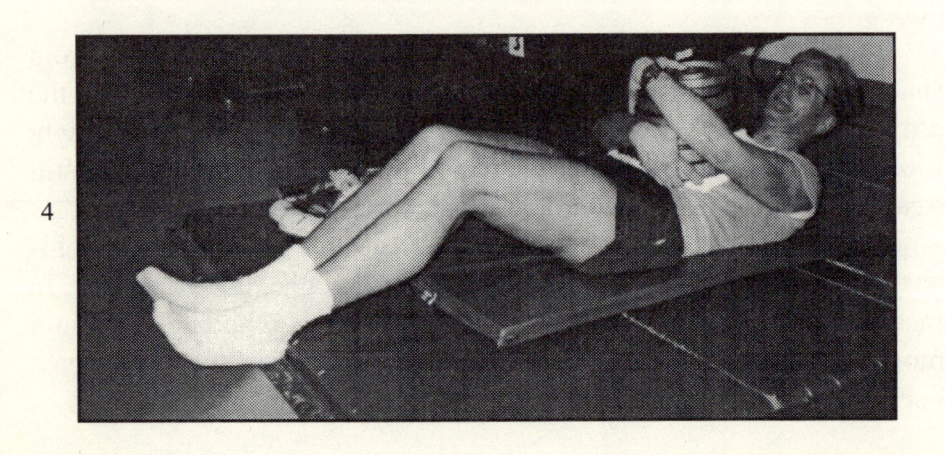

4

To speed things up, don't forget about the *multiplier effect*. When you do your sit-ups within the proper mental context, the outcome will be more pronounce given the same amount of effort.

You should notice some improvements in a month. If you stick to your game plan for another couple of months, even your friends who are heavier than you will admit that you look different—somehow. I am not saying that you should stop after three months or so. Once you achieved the results you wanted, and you got your weight down to an acceptable level, you still have to manage it. Instead of discontinuing your sit-ups completely, you can do them less frequently; but if you are going to take that route, also consider supplementing them with other forms of exercises.

This is when phase two kicks in. Now that you are really excited when you see that your abs are taking a different shape, you may even consider sculpting other parts of the body. There's always room for improvement. Depending on how much time you are willing to spare, you may want to try some of the following: building body mass with weights…gaining definition and improve your cardiovascular by taking part in rowing, swimming, bicycling, dance lessons, martial arts…toning your muscles by doing aerobics, isometrics, Pilates, or even walking at a brisk pace…realigning your posture by doing Pilates, et cetera."

"What did Michael do at that stage?"

"Losing all that weight encouraged him to try other things. He started rowing and cycling. When he was young, he cycled recreationally. 'I didn't get invited to do much of anything else because of my size,' he pointed out. 'My grandmother lived 15 miles away, and I had frequently rode to her place and back. Years later, I bought a good 10 speed. But I gave it up and did not cycle from 1986 to 1994.'

But in May of 1994, he took his old 10 speed out of the shed on his acreage and rode about 100 km. He then started commuting to work. He bought a better 10 speed in 1995 and commuted 100 times.

It was during one of those commutes that he met up with a 'racing cyclist'. He asked him if he was in a race club. He said, 'No, I don't think I am good enough.' He looked at him and said, 'Oh you are good enough— and you are riding a tank!' Michael made the decision then to join a club.

He joined the Edmonton Veterans Cycling Association. It was around that time when he took his cycling more serious and purchased a third bike—a Marinoni with Ultegra 600 specs. He took part in his first race—a 15 km time trial. 'I pedalled like mad without an aero bar or fancy wheels and ended up with the fastest time in my bracket.'

'Now, I am doing 15 km and 40 km time trials, road races, intra-provincial races, 'criteriums', and 'hillies'. I won a silver medal at one event in Drumheller, Alberta. I also won a bronze medal for the full year results in my class for time trials.'

His weight kept dropping. He was down to 190 pounds in April of 1994. By May, he was down to 180 pounds; by June, he was down to 170 pounds; by July, he was down to 160 pounds; and by August, he reached a low of 148 pounds which was a bit on the lean side for his 5'11" frame. During that period, he kept doing his sit-ups—as much as 1000 a day.

After he lost all that weight, he began to wonder about the loose skin around his face and body. 'People were beginning to think that I had AIDS or something.' he laughed.

That was when he joined a fitness club and began experimenting with weights. He tackled it with the same passion as his sit-ups. The weights helped him to gain some definition. 'Usually a good cyclist has a lean upper body, but my old cycling jersey became too tight, and it strangles my arms,' he pointed out.

Nevertheless, the weights improved his cycling by giving him more stamina to cover longer distances. He attributes it to the increase in the strength of his legs. He could leg press 1035 pounds and do 3 reps of 25's.

He also added more variety to his sit-ups. 'I do benching, reverse crunches, side pulls, leg lifts... Instead of hooking my ankles under a support, it's more challenging if I just let them dangle. It was much harder to do. But once I got the hang of it, I was able to climb back up to the number of repetitions that I used to do the old way.'

Besides doing sit-ups, cycling, and weights, he took advantage of everyday activities. He became interested in walking. He built up his pace until he could walk for an hour during most lunch hours. He also maintains four acres of land, four horses, and the usual 'farm work'. 'It's quite physical and does provide a variety to my exercise program,' he said.

At the moment, he is devoting more time to develop his legs for cycling. 'My new goal is to complete the famous cycling event: the Paris-Brest-Paris. It's held every four years. You must ride 1250 km in no more than 90 hours.'

With a proper diet and exercise, he's now back to 165 lb. In his mind, that seems to be ideal—if not perfect, since he is always striving for perfection. But it's a far cry from the image of the person he used to be. He still keeps his 'before' photo to remind himself of the horror of it all."

11

Playing The Part

"I don't know—" you said. Your doubts were starting to get the better part of you again. "I don't think I can do that many sit-ups."

"But that was Michael's way of doing it. He had increased his sit-ups immediately, and he kept doing that during the first three months—he did not resort to weight plates until later. Not only that, he increased them a lot. He resorted not just to the *intensity* of his sit-ups but also to their *frequency*—the number of times he does them. When the *multiplier effect* came into play, it boosted more and more of his *physical intensity* because he kept increasing his repetitions.

I am not saying that you have to resort to such extreme measures. What I want to emphasize by citing Michael as an example is that you have to be serious. If you are committed one day and not the next, it's not going to work. You have to keep at it.

It's possible to have a strong mental commitment without citing your affirmation or mission statement and without resorting to visualization. But not everyone can be as determined as Michael. According to him, it was 'pure determination'."

"Is that another way of bringing about the *multiplier effect*?"

"Yes, it's possible to assume the role that you want to play without depending on encouragement, short term results, or the right frame of mind. But for the majority of us, we need all the help we can get before we can start playing the part.

Remember, everyone starts at a different *intensity* level. That's why losing weight is so difficult. You cannot give someone a prepackaged program. You have to attend to each individual case.

If you can start with a bang, that's fine—but there's also the question of keeping up with the pace. And even if your are certain that you could, you can still reinforce it.

You want to make sure that the part you play is not just at the physical level. Having the proper *mental intensity* (the *intensity* of your visualization and your *intention*) can make a big difference in controlling the amount of calories you consume as well as getting rid of excess calories. It does this by reprogramming the way you think both consciously and subconsciously.

It all depends on the sort of information you feed into your thoughts. Sometimes you don't have to say it in so many words. Like right now for instance—you feel that it will probably not work for you. Then that sort of thinking determines the role that you are going to play. And so far you are playing the same part over and over again. You have to rewrite the script."

"But I've been very active over the years. Why didn't that make any difference?"

"If you happen to adopt the wrong attitude during all that time, then you are struggling with two opposing forces. Suppose that on the one hand, you feed your *mental intensity* with discouragement and doubts about your ability to change; and on the other, you are trying to change by engaging in the *physical intensity* of your exercises. Your *mental intensity* will likely win. Although you were determined enough to carry out your physical tasks, you were mentally acting out the wrong part. If you were mentally acting out the wrong part—like not caring about what you were eating, how often you ate, et cetera, then your body becomes less receptive to the desired physical changes."

"So you're saying that even if you are determined, it can still work against you?"

"Yes. If your determination is only at the physical level, you will then just go through the motions without adopting the proper *mental intensity*."

"Other than doing sit-ups, how else can I acquire the *proper mental intensity*?"

"I suggest that you start repeating your affirmation not just when you are working out but also at different times of the day—and hold the proper mental image of yourself at the same time. Your body will become receptive to your *intention* and your *visualization* all day. It's like acting out the new YOU around the clock.

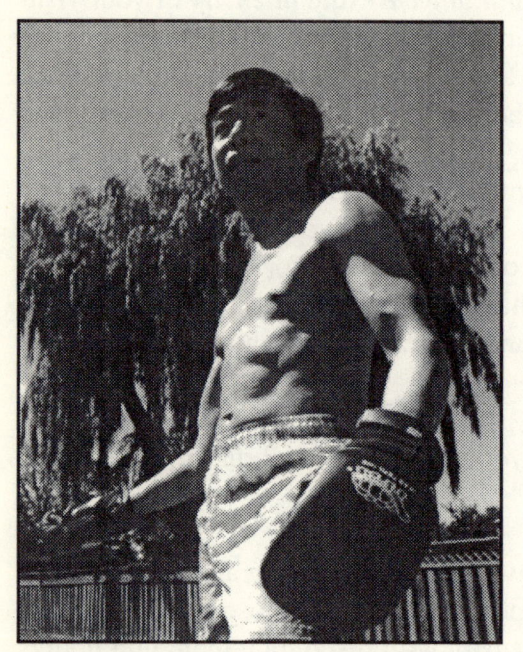

But this does not mean you can skip your sit-ups. When you increase the frequency of your visualization and affirmation, you are actually increasing the effect of the *multiplier* since your body will become more responsive to your sit-ups.

In other words, you are getting your abs ready (actually more than ready) to be molded. But if you do nothing else, your body will not take the proper shape. You may lose some weight and change your profile to a certain extent since 'playing the part' implies that you are activating your conscious and subconscious mind to regulate your habits and internal functions of your body. But in order to fine tune this approach, the *intensity factor* must also come into play; and that means doing your sit-ups.

Also, get a picture of the kind of 'washboard abs' that you want to have and paste it in front of you when you do your routine if you find that helpful.

To get over the illusion that you are not making any progress, resist being a scale watcher. The scale is not an accurate indicator of how much fat you have lost or need to lose. It's more of a reminder of how much fat you have. Get rid of it. Your belt is a better yardstick. It can tell you what the scale can't; you will know how much your waist has shrunken by the indentations made by the buckle.

The other reason for hiding your scale is that if you don't, you will be strictly thinking about losing weight as opposed to fat, and that can get you into all sorts of trouble.

Figure 5 in the handout I gave you is a picture of me just before my national competition. I only lost 1 pound even though I was still about 9 pounds heavier than the year before. However, I still lost 3 inches off my waist mainly by doing sit-ups and keeping a positive attitude. But if those 9 pounds of excess weight were not in the form of fat, what did it consisted of? Answer: muscle. I replaced the 9 pounds of fat I had with muscle.

If you find that you are losing weight without hardly making a dent in your cache of fat, you know something is wrong. You will know that you are losing fat if you just refer to the notches in your belt, your dress or pant size, or to your profile in front of mirror—although the latter may be a bit deceiving after a big meal because your stomach tends to bulge and will retain that shape for a couple of hours.

Imagine what would happen if I went strictly by the scale and was not aware that I had converted those 9 pounds into muscle and thought that they were still fat. What do you think my overall definition would look like if I went all out to get rid of those 9 pounds of muscle—which I thought was fat?"

"It's a scary thought," you admitted.

12

Other Ways To Speed Things Up

"I hope I will see some fast results."

"Although it's fast compared to most other methods, it's not going to be in terms of days or weeks. This is not a crash diet program."

"I realize that. My cousin was on one of those, and it didn't work. But she did lose a lot of weight during the first couple of weeks," you recalled.

"There is a difference between losing weight and getting rid of excess fat. When people lose weight in a hurry, what they are really trimming are the things their bodies need: water, glycogen, antibodies, enzymes, protein…
When you are depriving your body of its primary source of fuel—which is carbohydrate—by not eating, it will be short of glucose. It has to manufacture it from existing material by grabbing protein from your muscle tissue.
The real danger of going on a crash diet is that you will lose muscle as well as fat. Muscle is more dense than fat, and that's what actually registers on the scale as a loss. You may even lose more muscle than fat if your body gets the wrong signal and thinks you are starving yourself. It will slow your metabolism down to the point of conserving your body fat at all cost.

I want to make it clear that I am not telling you to cut back on your regular meals—although you may have to do something about your snacking if it is supplying you with more calories than you need; I will talk about this in a moment.

You need to be properly fuelled because you are trying to boost your existing activity in phase one, and later you will use the same approach to increase your overall activity in phase two. And I don't just mean doing sit-ups, aerobics, and resistance training; I will also elaborate on this topic later.

If you plan to increase your overall activity to boost you metabolism while restricting your body from its source of fuel, it is like trying to drive with the gas pedal fully depressed while ignoring the warning from your fuel gauge. Your engine will be spitting and sputtering; and eventually, it will stall.

Where do you think your body will get its fuel if you don't give it any?"

"You don't mean…" you said when you thought back on all those lunches you skipped.

"Exactly. It will probably eat your muscles up at a faster rate than you can build them.

An overall exercise routine is something for you to consider later. What you are going to do first is to gradually ease into it—not just going through the physical motions but also taking part in the mental aspect of 'slashing your weight and trimming your abs'.

You will start your routine with side sit-ups. If you did not do any form of exercise for ages, then side sit-ups are a comfortable way to start. Most people find that they are easy to do. When you tackle the front sit-ups or front 'crunches' next, your number of repetitions will likely drop. By the time you get around to your reverse 'crunches', don't be surprise if you end up doing even less. But that is OK since 'crunches' are harder to do.

When you are well into your routine, the pendulum will start swinging the other way; and it will not be unusual to double, triple, or even quadruple the average number of sit-ups that you did during the first week. After a month or so, like I said, you can start thinking about increasing the load instead of your 'reps'.

But before you do that, I am going to give you a few more options which are just as effective:

1. You can also change the order of your sit-ups by doing the more difficult ones first—and this is another way of increasing your load *internally*. You can start with your front 'crunches', then go to your reverse 'crunches', and save the side sit-ups for last.

By the time you do your side sit-ups, you will end up doing less, but that is OK; you are way ahead in the total amount of calories you burn. You will warm up quicker since it takes more effort to do extra front 'crunches' and reverse 'crunches'. You are ensuring that the fat burning process kicks in faster; and the faster it kicks in, the higher it will peak during the short duration of your workout. This is essential because fat burns slowly.

2. If you are having trouble fulfilling your quota of 'crunches', you also have the option of doing them in sets—which is actually another way of increasing your 'reps'.

Let's say that you are able to do a total of 100 side sit-ups, but it takes too much time before you 'feel' that you are benefiting from them. So you decide to change the order of your sit-ups. But suppose that although you can do more front 'crunches', you are almost running on 'empty' when you attempt your reverse 'crunches'. When you did what you could with the side sit-ups, you did not even pass the 5 minute mark.

One way to get around this problem is to do 2 or 3 sets of reverse 'crunches' instead of just 1 set. Your may do 10 repetitions during your first set, and your may only do 5 on your next 2 sets. But that's 20 repetitions altogether. You are taking a break between each set, and you will find that you will end up with a higher count.

If you find that you are still finishing up your routine before 5 minutes, you can also break up your front 'crunches' into sets."

"What if you are still falling behind?"

"Then go back to your reverse 'crunches'. Use them to fill up any gaps you might have."

"Why reverse 'crunches'?"

"They are easier on your lower back. When it comes to doing one or two more sets beyond your comfort level, it's a logical precaution to take."

"You are actually taking a rest between sets, and that allows you to do more," you realized.

"Yes, and the interruption allows you to catch your breath. A lot of people forget to breathe properly when they work out. The worse you can do is to hold your breath. Oxygen is a necessary ingredient in the breakdown of fat. The body needs oxygen before it can burn fat, so don't forget to breathe deeply when you do your sit-ups. Inhale when you sit back, and exhale when you sit up. Continue to breathe deeply between sets.

Another way to speed up your progress is to do your exercises the same time each day. Your body will adjust to that schedule. And try to do it when you are energetic. In my case, that is the first thing in the morning.

Sometimes I even do them about an hour before I go to sleep. I would just do one type of sit-up; in my case, that happens to be the front 'crunch' since I don't do enough of them. Another reason why I just stick to one type of sit-up at night is because I'm not that motivated. If I had to do the whole routine, I might skip the idea despite the fact that it only takes 5 minutes.

Don't go through the movement nonstop for 5 minutes. Do them in sets. Notice here that you are combining two different techniques to speed things up: you are doing them in sets, and you are doing double time by doing your favourite sit-up at night as well as during the day.

Don't go to sleep immediately after you finish your sets. Allow yourself to wind down a bit first. Your metabolic rate, however, will tend to remain higher by the time you go to bed. It is like burning extra calories while you are sleeping."

"Can I try some of the sit-ups?" you asked. All this talk about speeding things up made you want to get right into it.

"Sure," I replied as I took you over to one of the mobile mats.

"Let's rock and roll," you said with conviction as you quickly flipped to the exercise section of the workbook I gave you.

"The sit-ups are self explanatory. Remember, you only have to choose four."

"Any four?"

"Any four that target the sides and upper and lower regions of your abdomen," I confirmed. "And don't forget about your mental attitude when you do them."

"The *multiplier*," you recalled.

"Exactly."

13

Getting On Your Butt

"When you do the following sit-ups, do not rush through them. It is not how fast, but how many that counts. I've already condensed the time you will spend by substituting the duration of your workout with its *intensity*. If you cut any more corners, you may save more time—but you may also end up saving something else: the bulk of your fat.

It does not mean, however, that you should do them so slow that you end up straining yourself. Aim for a steady rhythm instead. In other words, you are not running a 5 minute mile; you are doing it for 5 minutes.

Another reason why I tell people to stick to a 5 minute routine in the beginning is that there is the tendency to quit if they do not ease themselves into the *duration* of the routine as well as its *intensity*—even if it's only for 5 minutes. Once you whipped yourself into shape, that's another story. When you start seeing some short term results, that's enough to entice you to go for 10 minutes—or even 15. But because of the *intensity factor* behind how I want you to do your sit-ups, it's not necessary to do them longer than that. So, are you ready?"

"All set," you said as you got on the mat. You were eager to try them out on your own.

"All right, go to it," I signalled you to start.

SIDE SIT-UP

Let's tackle the obliques by starting with sit-ups against your right side:

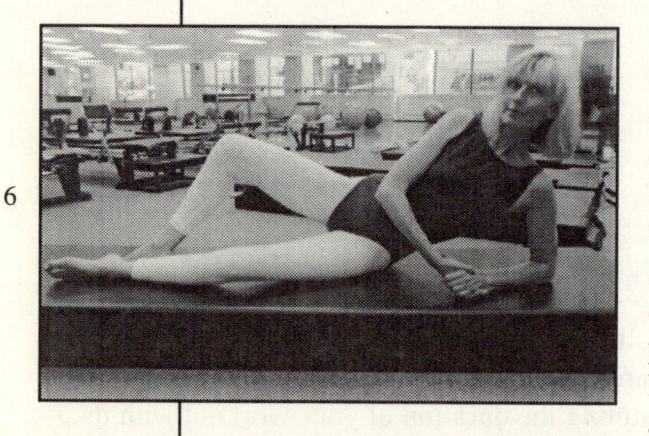

1. Sit on your left buttock and against the side of your left leg which is drawn up close to you. Draw up the right leg until the bottom of your foot is flat on the mat, and your right knee is pointing upwards. Your left forearm is resting against the mat, and the weight of your upper body is on it. Clasp your left hand onto your right. See figure 6.

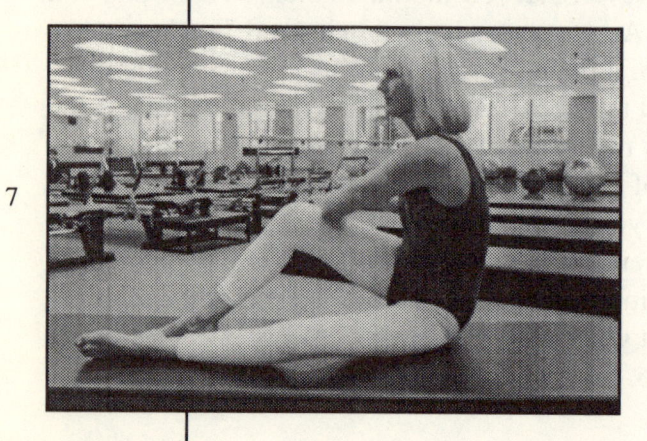

2. Sit up and twist your waist until your left elbow touches your right knee. See figure 7.

3. Next, turn facing your left again and go back down only halfway. Do not rest on your left forearm. *You are always carrying a constant load.* See figure 8.

4. Then twist your waist and sit up at the same time as in step 2, et cetera. Repeat the same movement on your opposite side against your left obliques. In this case, you will sit up and turn and touch your left knee.

Getting On Your Butt

You twist and turn because that is what your obliques were designed for. Once you strengthen those muscles, you will improve the efficiency of their tasks.

Do a few on each side of your body first to get used to the load. Refrain from getting carried away; otherwise, you will feel it the next day. If you can only do a total of 10 the first day, that's OK. But strive to gradually increase your "reps". If you have difficulty going through the movements, grab hold of your raised knee with one hand for leverage. Allow the other arm to swing freely to assist in lifting you off the mat.

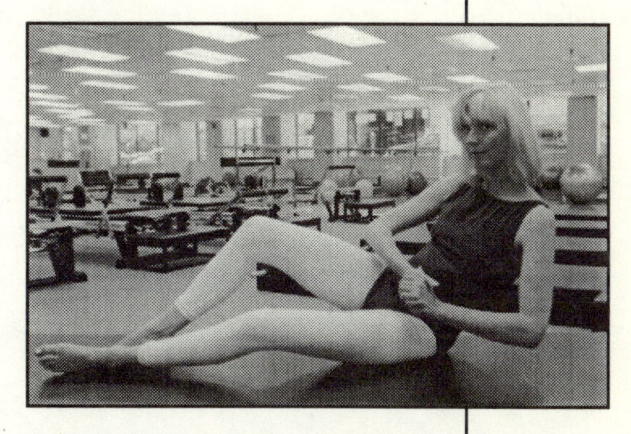

FRONT CRUNCH

We will concentrate on the upper abs first with my version of a front sit-up or "crunch":

1. Lift your feet off the floor and draw your knees up close to your face. Your lower legs are horizontal to the floor. Cross your ankles to improve your stability. Support the back of your head with your hands. Do not clasp your fingers. See figure 9. If you cannot keep your legs up, prop them up on something.

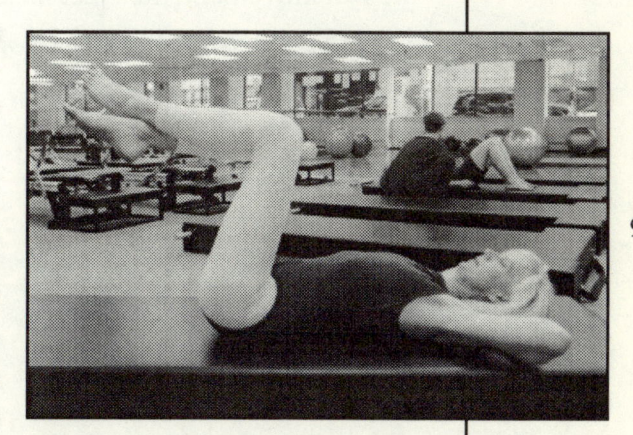

2. Sit up and touch your knees with your elbows as in figure 10. If that is difficult at first, draw your knees closer to your face or come as close to your knees as possible. Do not pull your head forward. Your hands are only supporting your head. The length of your arms act as a gauge to tell you how far you should sit up. Your lower back is still resting on the mat, so there should be almost no pressure against it.

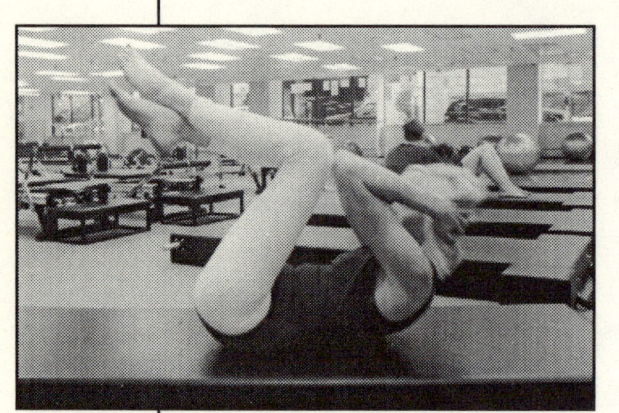

3. Then go back down halfway. Do not rest your head or upper back on the mat. Your hands are cradling your head again. *You are always carrying a constant load.* See figure 11.

4. Then sit up and touch your knees with your elbows as in step 2, et cetera. If you have difficulty going through the full movement, then just raise yourself up a quarter of the way. Then work your way up higher as your abs get stronger.

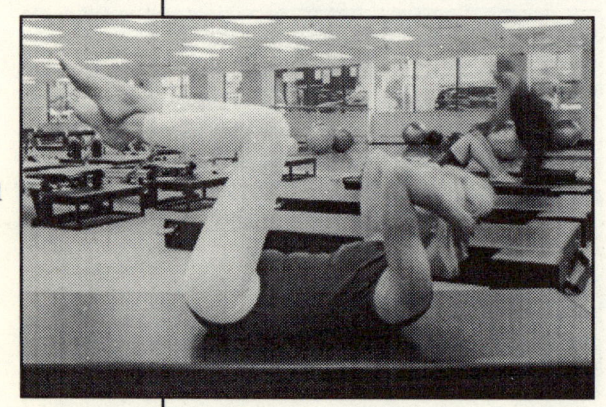

TOE-TOUCH CRUNCH

Once you get used to the initial load that you imposed on your abs, here's another variation that's a bit more challenging:

1. Lie flat on your back and raise both your legs straight up until they are perpendicular to the floor as in figure 12.

2. Sit up and touch your toes. Your lower back is still resting on the mat. If you have difficulty doing that at first, come as close as possible to your toes, or bend your knees slightly, or tilt your legs towards you a bit. See figure 13.

3. Then go back down halfway. Do not rest your head or upper back on the mat. Tuck your chin forward a bit to ease the strain on your neck. *You are always carrying a constant load.* See figure 14. (If you find this hard to do at first, go all the way down each time.)

It's the vertical movement as oppose to a lateral one that makes this sit-up difficult. You will really begin to feel it at first even if you are well versed in performing the regular "crunches".

REVERSE CRUNCH

Now let's tackle the lower abs with the "reverse crunch":

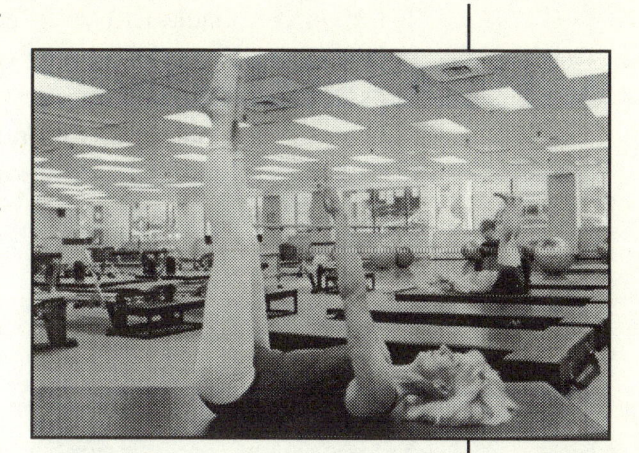

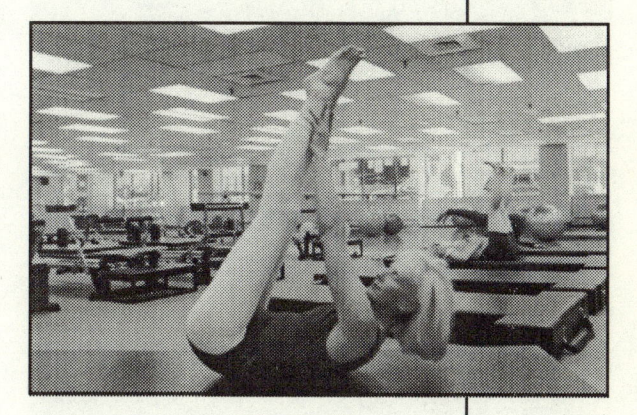

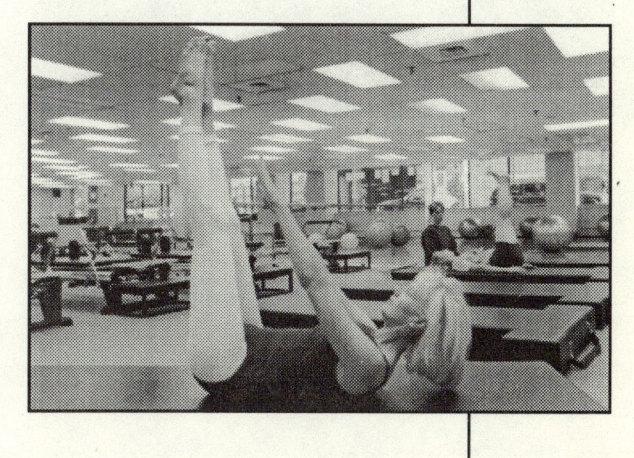

12

13

14

1. Lie on your back. Lift your feet off the floor and draw your knees up. Your lower legs are horizontal to the floor. Cross your ankles to improve your stability. Rest your arms with your palms down on the mat beside you. See figure 15.

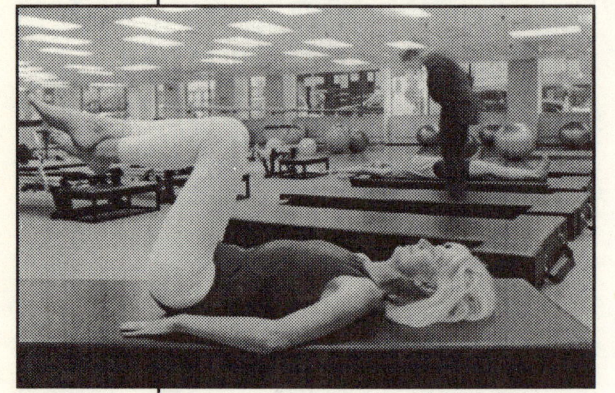

2. Raise your rear off the mat as in figure 16. You do not have to raise it high.

3. Next, go back down (all the way down). Then repeat.

Once your abs becomes more developed, you can modify the "reverse crunch" by resting your arms on your chest to refrain from using them as leverage. That makes it a bit harder, but it's well worth the effort.

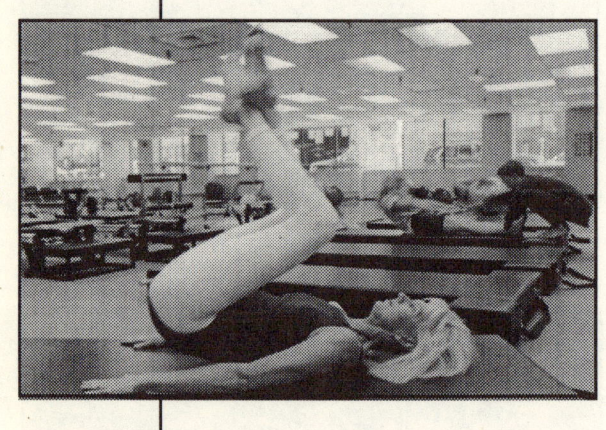

14

The Good Old Ab Bench

I was surprise you were still going at a decent pace when I went over to see how you were doing. "How do you feel?"

"No problem," you said without slowing down.

"OK, stop for a minute," I said with some concern. "Let's not get too far ahead on the first day."

"But I can still do more."

"It's better if you ease into it," I reminded. "Pay attention to how you feel tomorrow. If it's not too stressful, then increase your 'reps'. You are probably all excited about doing something new on the first day. When your adrenaline is high, you probably wouldn't feel any pain—if you are in pain—until the next day.
Let's shift gears for a minute and do a quick review: you must increase the number of repetitions after your body adapts to the initial quantity you imposed on it. I don't think you will have any problem with that. But after you increased your 'reps' several times, you might want to consider increasing the load if you are doing a lot of 'reps' without 'feeling' it or without getting the sort of benefit you would expect in proportion to the effort that you put in.
One way to increase the load, as I have said, is by doing your sit-ups in a different order. It will take more effort because you are doing the

front and reverse 'crunches' first. Those are the types of sit-ups that require you to displace more weight. If you cannot do as many 'reps' as you would like given the increase in your load, don't forget the option of doing your 'crunches' in sets. The break between each set allows you to take a short rest, and you will end up doing more sit-ups. Now, I'm going to show you another way to increase the load."

"I'm all for it."

"The ab bench is another way of creating a heavier load without resorting to external weights; you are increasing the load *internally*. The steeper you set the incline, the heavier the load. You are displacing more of your weight as the bench approaches the vertical position. The angle of the bench also gives you a wider range of movement; you can lean farther back, and this will make you do more work.

You do not need an ab board. But if you do not find the floor exercises challenging enough after your abs get more developed, then you may consider it as an option. Its appeal is overshadowed by the flood of high-tech exercise equipment and gut-busting aids. But I think it is still the most effective piece of equipment around as far as 'slashing your weight and trimming your abs' is concerned.

If you are good at carpentry, you can construct one yourself; it will save you a bundle of money. A piece of plank 1 ft. x 4 ft. will do nicely. Add a piece of 2 X 2 going across the length of it—about a foot and a half or so from the top for your legs to cradle over. Lean it against a crate or some similar object. Besides providing the proper angle, it also serves as an ankle constraint; all you have to do is to place the balls of your feet against it, and you are all set to go. It might also be a good idea to add another 2 X 2 onto the underside of the plank—a bit ahead of the first piece—so that it latches against the crate to keep the board from slipping.

An easier way to do it is to lean the plank against a large bag of rice—a 25 pound bag or 50 pound bag; and that's all there is to it. You don't have to make, cut, or hammer away at anything. To get a good foothold, spread your knees apart and dig your heels into the bag until they catch the edge of the board.

Although this set up is great for your front and reverse 'crunches', side sit-ups will be awkward to do. To get around this problem, do your 'crunches' on the ab board first and finish up your side sit-ups on the floor. You will still feel it because most of your energy will be expended doing the harder variety of sit-ups.

A makeshift ab bench—or 'ab board' as I will also call it to remind you that it can be home-made—may not look expensive, but it will 'feel' just like the real thing."

"Do you have one here?" you asked.

"Yep, in the next room."

"Is it the 'real thing'?"

"Once you get on it, you wouldn't notice the difference."

You went back to the exercise section of your workbook and continued from where you left off. I got the hint that you wanted to be left alone again.

SIDE SIT-UP ON THE AB BENCH

Let's start with a few sit-ups on the ab bench for your right obliques:

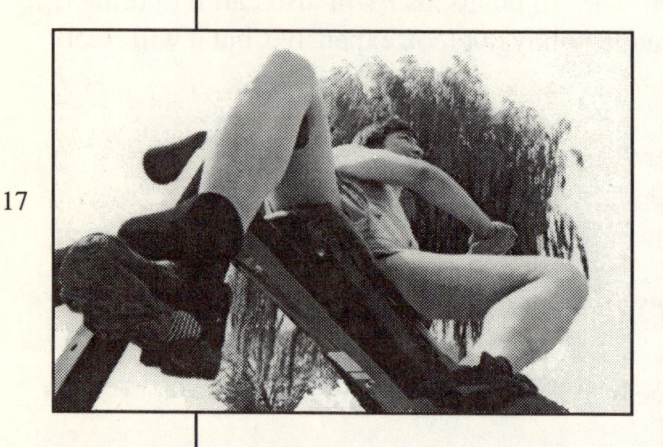

17

1. Hook your right leg over the roller and the right foot under the left ankle constraint. Your left foot is touching the floor slight ahead of you. When you turn to the left, you are isolating the right obliques for this exercise. Lean back—but not too far back. Your left forearm does not touch the board, and you are not resting your body against it. *You are always carrying a constant load against your obliques.* See figure 17.

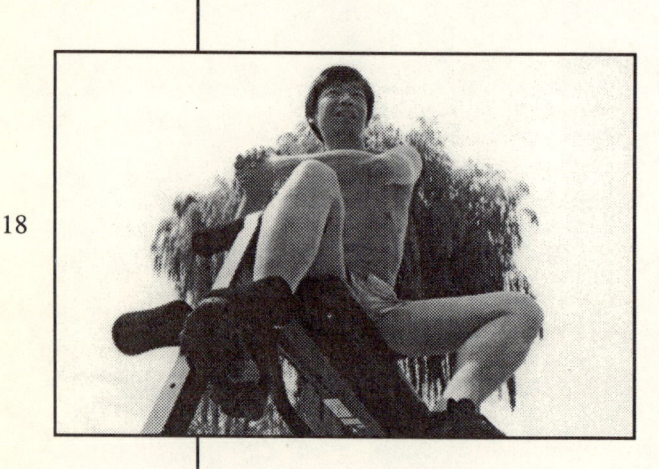

18

2. Clasp both your hands together. Sit up and twist your body clockwise to the right until you are facing the front. Continue twisting until you can almost touch your right knee with your left elbow. It is not necessary to strain yourself to touch it. If you stop inches away from it, that's fine since your hip flexors will be taking over anyway once you go past vertical. See figure 18.

Doing this exercise on the ab board allows you a wider range of movement. The more you turn sideways and the farther you lean backwards, the greater the distance you have to cover when you sit up. You will end up imparting a heavier load to your obliques. This side to side and up and down movement on the ab board could very well be the answer for your bulging sides.

Repeat the above movements against your left obliques by hooking your left leg over the right roller and the left foot under the right ankle constraint. Then go through the above movements on that side. See figures 19 and 20.

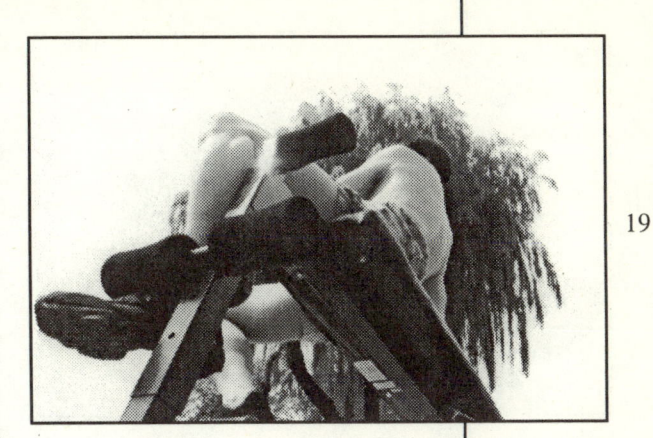

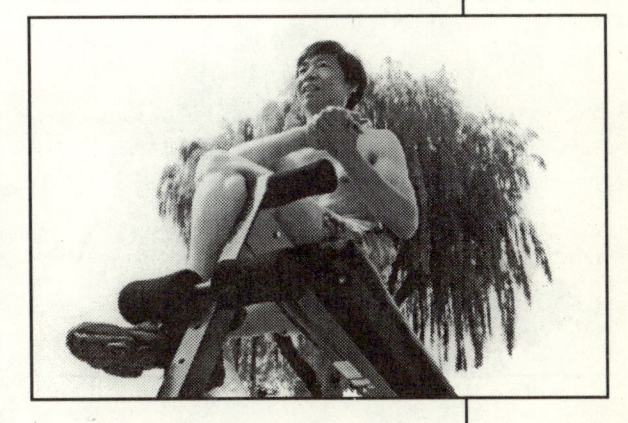

FRONT CRUNCH ON THE AB BENCH

The front "crunch" on the ab bench is done almost the same way as you would do it on the floor. The only difference is that you go through a wider range of movement, and you are displacing a heavier load due to the angle of the board. The steeper you set the angle, the more weight you have to displace.

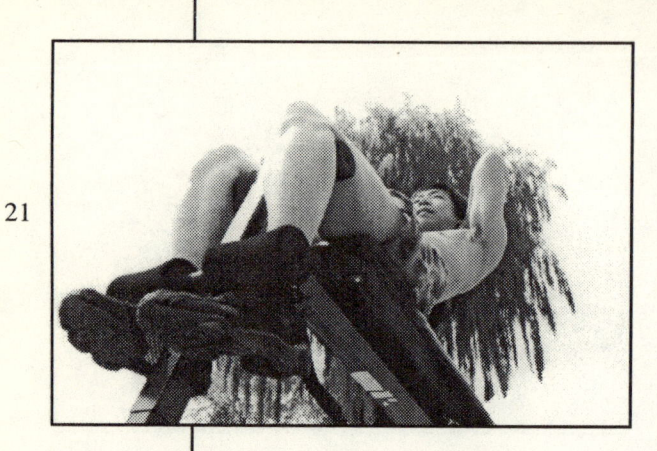

1. Hook both of your feet under the ankle constraints. Then lean back. You do not have to go all the way down on the board. See figure 21.

Support your head with your hands. Do not clasp your fingers to avoid the tendency of yanking against your head when you sit up.

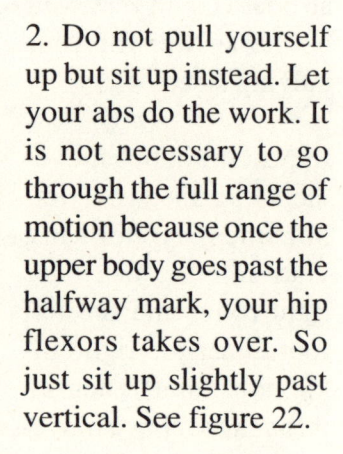

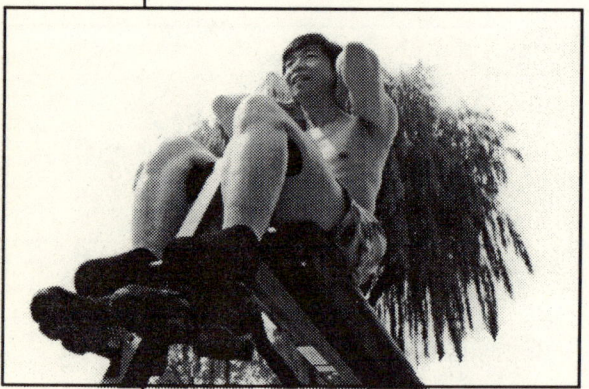

2. Do not pull yourself up but sit up instead. Let your abs do the work. It is not necessary to go through the full range of motion because once the upper body goes past the halfway mark, your hip flexors takes over. So just sit up slightly past vertical. See figure 22.

If you are having trouble leaning back far enough, you can grip the edges or the sides of the board and ease yourself back. The length of your arms act as a gauge to control how far back you go.

When your abs become stronger, support your head with your hands and lean farther back. It is harder to maintain a constant load since more of your weight is imparted to your abs instead of your arms. But once you get the hang of it, it is an excellent way of trimming and toning your abs; they are benefiting from the downstroke almost as much as from the upstroke. The fluctuation between maintaining the load when you lean back and displacing the load when you lean forward will burn more calories.

REVERSE CRUNCH ON THE AB BENCH

Doing the reverse "crunches" on the ab bench is almost similar to the way that you would do it on the floor. Again, you are lifting a heavier load due to the angle of the board. But because you are in the supine position, there is less pressure on your lower back compared to the other types of sit-ups. If I wanted to do lots of "sets", I would start with this type of sit-up. Then I would wind down with the front "crunch", and then finally to the side sit-up.

1. Turn around and face the foot of the ab board. Lie down on the head rest and grab the upper corners or the rollers with both your hands.

2. Raise your legs and bend your knees towards you. Cross your ankles for stability and for a bit of leverage.

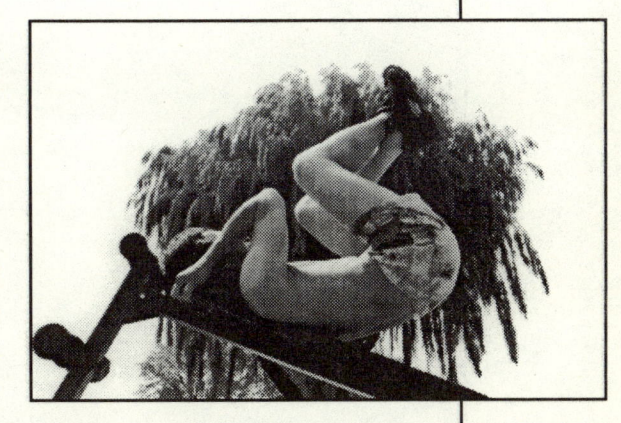

3. Then raise your rear off the bench. It does not have to be high. See figure 23.

4. Then go back down until your lower back rests on the board. Your lower legs will drop a bit, but try to keep your feet off the floor. Your knees will likely be pointing up as you try to keep your feet from touching down. From this position, raise your rear off the bench again.

5. Continue in a rocking motion.

As with the floor exercises, once you get used to doing the side sit-ups, you may want to change the order of your routine by starting off with the "crunches" first. This is particularly effective on the ab bench. You will be experiencing a heavier load from the change in the order that you do your sit-ups plus the load created by the angle of the bench.

15

Applying An External Load

"How are you doing?" I asked as I went back to check on you.

"Very intense," you said as you laid motionless on the ab board.

"It's harder when you do your sit-ups at an angle. But don't worry, you'll get used to it. You're doing find. You're off to a good start. Let's take a break."

"Could I combine some of the sit-ups on the ab bench with those done on the floor?"

"Sure, if you can do it."

"I think I can do my side sit-ups on the ab bench and the 'crunches' on the floor."

"That's a good idea. If you cannot get a hold of an ab bench—and you do not feel like making one yourself—another way to increase the load is by applying an *external* load. That means you are actually going to carry an object like a weight plate, a dumbbell, or a bag of rice (which is safer and distributes the weight more evenly).

The way Michael did it, if you recall, is by placing weight plates on his chest. It's like pumping weights: suppose you got used to heaving a barbell set to the point where your third set does not feel much different from your fourth set; then it might be a good idea to add some more weight plates. Otherwise, you are limiting the development of your muscles.

And when you get used to the load, you can start to increase the number of 'reps' again. Of course, there is a limit to the number of repetition you can do and to how much weights you can add. You have to use your best judgment. Always keep in mind that you do not want to add too much stress to your lower back."

"Wouldn't I get a sore neck from doing this kind of sit-up?"

"You can avoid that problem by tucking your chin in and, whenever possible, cradling your head. This applies to any type of front sit-up.

A few words of caution: I suggest that you omit carrying any sort of external weights when you do your side sit-ups. It creates too much strain on your lower back—especially when you twist.

Also forget about carrying an external load when you perform your reverse 'crunches'. It is awkward, and it can also be too strenuous on your lower back. It is safer to lift an external load when you are doing a front sit-up because your lower back is still on the floor throughout the range of movement.

When you reach this stage, I am assuming that you are beginning your order of sit-ups with the front 'crunch', and that the harder variety of sit-ups are not offering you much of a challenge.

Maintain the same order when you decide to add an external load to your front sit-up. It should give you a faster warm up—due to the external load plus the load from the order you do your sit-ups.

This in turn allows the reverse 'crunch' and side sit-ups to be more effective as far as the fat burning process goes. Your muscles will tend to work harder to complete your routine."

"I'm curious how that feels," you said. You went over to the rack and fetched a dumbbell.

"I suggest you start with a single weight plate instead."

You thought about it for a moment and fetched a variety of weight plates. You were ready to go at it again.

FRONT CRUNCH WITH AN EXTERNAL LOAD

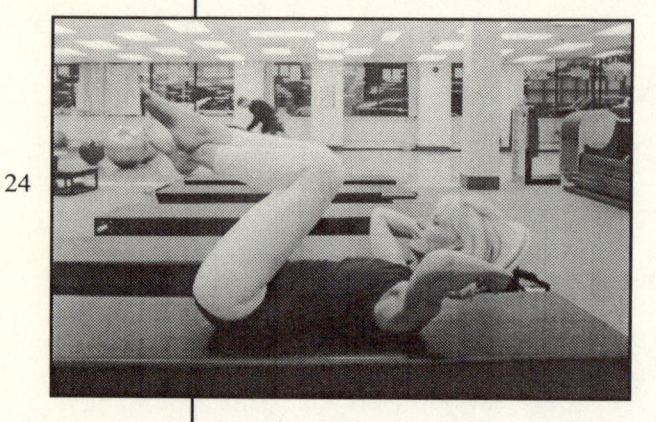

24

Hold the weight plate against the back of your head and perform your normal "crunches". Do not use the plate as leverage to pull yourself up. That will cause a lot of strain against your neck. Use your abs instead. See figure 24 and 25.

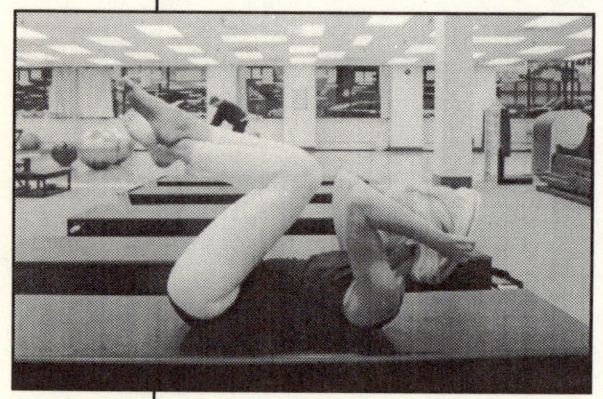

25

If you are using a dumbbell, hold the ends and press it against your chest. The palms of your hands are facing you. Sit up until the back of your hands touch your thighs. Spread your knees to allow the weight plates to pass through. If that is difficult to do at first, just touch your thighs with the weights plates instead of the back of your hands. See figures 26 and 27.

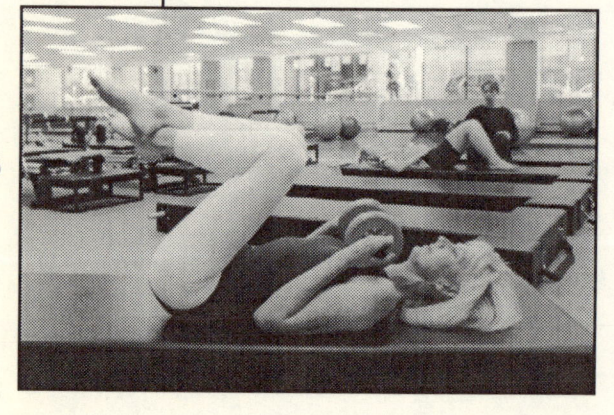

26

When you get used to the load, increase it; but think about safety first. Go slowly. If it does not seem to work, abandon the idea and wait until your abs are stronger.

Applying An External Load

Maybe some of you are tempted to try doing your "crunches" on the ab bench while carrying an external weight of some sort. If you can do it, fine. But do not overdo it. You are already imposing an extra load on your lower back due to the angle of the bench and to the wider range of movement.

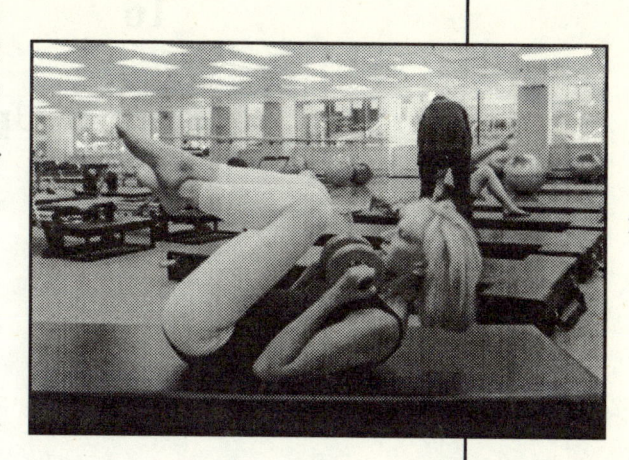

Also, when you are on the ab board, your lower back is raised when you are doing your front "crunches". It does not rest on the bench like the way it does when you do them on the floor.

The older you are, the disks between the vertebrae of your spine loses their elasticity. Too much downward pressure over an extended period of time, as in the case of excessive weight lifting, may compress them to the point where they will not regain their original shape.

16

Chalking It Up

"Here are some monthly charts," I said. I gave you enough to keep you going for three months—the average duration of my program.

"I have divided them into four parts. Record the number of sit-ups you do each day on your right obliques, left obliques, upper abs, and lower abs. The side sit-ups are for your obliques, the front 'crunches' are designed for the upper abs, and reverse 'crunches' are for the lower abs. Just concentrate on those four types of sit-ups during phase one.

The charts also play an important part in assisting you with your visualization. After a couple of months, you will become hazy about the amount of sit-ups that you are *capable* of doing. You may not think that it's anything worth bragging about; but if you kept track of how many you did each month, it can do wonders as far as visualizing the sort of results you want.

If you intend to do a total of 150 sit-ups a day, for example, that's 4500 sit-ups a month according to my 30 day a month chart. And that, in turn, adds up to an impressive 13,500 repetitions in three months. Ignore the extra days in the months that have more than 30 days. You can take a break. You deserve it.

And you can also measure your progress graphically on a line chart or a bar chart. You can divide the horizontal axis into weeks and the vertical axis into number of total sit-ups.

I am not saying that by the end of the third month, you will undergo an instant metamorphosis and shed your outer layer of unwanted fat.

Depending on your commitment and the shape that you are in, it's possible to see a difference a lot sooner."

"What if someone was struggling with a very tight schedule?" you asked with some concern.

"Then that person might have to wait a bit longer before there would be any noticeable results. Remember, fat burns slowly. It's impossible to get rid of it in a couple of weeks. If you listen to those who tell you otherwise, you will probably end up doing something drastic—like going on a crash diet of some sort. Then you will not just be losing fat when you lose weight. Most likely you will be losing something else that your body needs.

A safer way to speed up the program, as I have mentioned, is to start increasing the number of sit-ups that you do. You do not have to show an increase each day. But the faster you get around to it, the faster you will see results. And don't forget that at some point it's going to level off. That's OK if it represents your optimum performance.

The charts will help you keep your *intention* intact. If you are serious one day and not the next, or if you are only serious one week in a month, it will not work. And you will see how serious you are by checking your charts. If you see blotches of empty squares or a string of 5 or 10 sit-ups each day, you will know that the program is going to take awhile before it will work for you—if it is going to work at all."

"Are the charts themselves a motivating factor?"

"No doubt about it. It's like the 'high' that a jogger feels. But if your charts are properly maintained, you will feel it before as well as after you do your routine.

Try to come up with the desired number of sit-ups you want to do by the end of the first month, by the end of the second, and by the end of the third. Those targeted numbers of sit-ups are not cast in stone. You make adjustments as you go along. Some people progress slower while others will move along a little faster. By the end of the first month, you will have some idea of how much to increase or lower for the next month.

And by the end of the second month, you may want to do the same thing for the third month.

After the third month, you may not want to increase your 'reps' anymore. You may have reached your limit for the year. You may not even want to consider doing any other types of exercises. If that is what your body is telling you, that's OK. Listen to it. Again, like I said, there is no rush. Go slowly. Remember, you are burning fat."

17

Controlling Your Snacking Binges

"Another thing you have to do is cut your intake of snacks. The fat content in most snacks, especially junk food, is high. The kind of fat that you should be wary of is 'saturated' fat which is converted into cholesterol by your liver—especially LDL cholesterol.

There are two types of cholesterol: HDL or high density lipoproteins (the *good* type) and LDL or low-density lipoproteins (the *bad* type). Both of them together, from a fat standpoint, are neither good nor bad. They are rather *ugly* despite the fact that HDL cholesterol actually helps your body get rid of the LDL type of cholesterol which causes the build up of plaque on the walls of your arteries.

In other words, I don't recommend that you start increasing your doses of 'unsaturated' fat which contains HDL cholesterol. Unsaturated fat is still fat no matter how you look at it. But if you had to make a decision between saturated and unsaturated fat, go with the latter; for example, if you had to choose between lard and vegetable oil to fry your favourite dish, go with vegetable oil since unsaturated fat is found in vegetable products.

Total cholesterol levels less than 200mg/dL and LDL cholesterol level of less than 130mg/dL are deemed desirable.

All animal related foods contain cholesterol. If your snack included eggs, then you are stocking up on cholesterol. And if those eggs were used to make the apple pie which you had gulped down, then you are also loading up with saturated fats since a pie crust contains 3/4 to 1 cup of pure lard—some people use butter instead but it is just as bad since saturated fat, like cholesterol, is also found mainly in animal products. Whether you realized it or not, you have stockpiled stacks of calories from ingredients that are soaked with both cholesterol and saturated fat. And remember, your liver will convert the saturated fat from your apple pie into cholesterol, and that gets added to the cholesterol from your eggs."

"So you are often hit with a double whammy when you snack," you began to realize.

"Yes, because you tend to do it indiscriminately."

"How do I cut down?" you sounded a bit guilty.

"This is where your *intention* to lose weight comes into play."

"You mean my commitment to my affirmation?"

"Yes, and it's worthwhile to add a sentence or two to your affirmation about getting rid of your snacking habit. When you get rid of the *habit*, you can still snack. The only difference is that it is no longer a *habit*; and when it is no longer a *habit*, it will be easier for you to reduce your intake of snacks. I found that some of my students' *intention* to reduce their snacks merely meant snacking six times a day instead of seven. The *intention* is there, but so is the *habit*."

"Maybe their thoughts were not *intense* enough."

"That's right, and it should become easier to reduce your snacks when you start seeing some short term results and when you begin to realize that you are conforming to the image of the new YOU. Don't wait until you are in the second phase before you decide to do something about it. It'll be too late because you may never get to phase two. This is one case where garbage in does not equal garbage out. Most of it stays in.
Another way to break the *habit* is to get away from the environment that causes you to snack. If you are stuck at home with nothing to do all day, then snacking becomes more tempting.

Go on a vacation, a short trip, or a series of one day excursions. Join a club. Take classes. Get out of the house after dinner and go for a brisk walk. Go fishing—and by the way, fishing is one recreation where I can engage in all day without eating or feeling hungry."

"But I thought you said that starving yourself does not work."

"Your *intention* is different in this case: you just want to break the *habit* of snacking—not to starve yourself. If one of the ways to accomplish that is by not eating, there is a limit to how far you will go. Don't confuse a technique that helps you to abstain from overeating to a diet that's designed to reduce your normal intake of food.

Instead of relying on a single technique, it is more effective to combine them: like taking a course on fishing—believe it or not, there are courses like that. Once you attend a few classes, you will realize that you are doing several things: First, you are getting away from the factors that cause you to go on a snacking binge—like being glued in front of the TV. Second, you are becoming more active. And third, you are replacing an old habit with an interesting activity which does not involve snacking.

Once you modify your behaviour, then the conditions that caused you to snack should have less of an impact."

"Couldn't I just do my sit-ups more often?"

"You can't use exercise as an excuse to snack."

"But what about the *intensity factor*? Couldn't that take care of the accumulation of fat and cholesterol?"

"You can exercise until you are blue in the face, but the plaque formed by the LDL type of cholesterol will still linger around because it is not a fuel. You can't burn it off. You can only get rid of it by reducing your intake of saturated fat and foods that are high in cholesterol."

"Cutting my snacking habit is one thing, but I don't think I can completely cut out my snacking," you confessed.

"Then at least try managing it."

"What do you mean by managing it?"

"When you do snack, try to reduce the portions of your snack. In other words, instead of having two slices of apple pie, strive to settle for one piece; or instead of settling for an apple pie and ice cream, go with either the pie or the ice cream—not both. But this technique is only effective if you don't try to make up for it later on.

By managing it, you are doing two things:

1. It means that you are still striving to *totally* eliminate the habit. It may be an unrealistic goal at the moment, but at least the *intention* is there. And when you have the *correct intention*, your *amount* of snacking should dramatically decrease. It takes practise before you can get rid of the habit. It's similar to making a commitment to satisfy your quota of sit-ups; you begin in small spurts and work up instead of trying to acquire the will power to do it all at once.

2. Even if you completely cut your snacking, you still need the will power to manage those special occasions when you do go all out. Having some control here is critical. The last thing you want is to rekindle an old habit and provoke the chance of a relapse. However, I still treat myself to a snack now and then. I do not starve myself.

Sometimes I even tell people to snack occasionally instead of substituting their snack—along with their breakfast and lunch—with one big meal everyday."

"Are you saying that sometimes snacking now and then is a good practise to build that control?"

"That's right. Once I had a client who could not eliminate her snacking habit regardless of how hard she tried. We then decided that instead of struggling to give up snacking, she would become more selective. With practise, she was able to pause and think instead of instinctively reaching out for something. By the very act of choosing what to snack and deciding when to snack, she gained control not only of the *amount* she ate but also the *frequency* or how often she ate.

By allowing yourself to snack, you are not fighting with yourself all the time. If you keep telling yourself, 'I'm not going to snack, I'm not going to snack, I'm not going to snack...' You will likely end up snacking. Then you will feel guilty and hate yourself for giving in. When you constantly repeat to yourself what you are not going to do, you are inadvertently summoning up the very *habit* that you are struggling with—a *habit* that has conditioned and brainwashed you for years. Since you keep bringing it up, it acts as a constant reminder.

It makes a difference if you said instead, 'I'm going to lighten up on my snacks'."

"You are not challenging the demons that cause you to snack incessantly," you concluded.

"That's right. Once you included a statement in your affirmation that you will 'lighten up', it implies that you will try to be more selective in your snacking and that you are aiming to reduce its *amount* and *frequency*.

Some of my clients told me that when they tried this technique, they were satisfied with the degree of control they had over their snacking binges. It made very little difference, in terms of their daily calorie intake, whether they were snacking or not."

"Interesting," you commented. "All this talk about food is making my stomach growl."

"Let's go out for lunch," I offered.

"I don't usually have lunch."

"In your case, I suggest you should eat something. I know that it will be hard at first—probably just as hard as reducing your snacks; but one of the ways to reduce your snacks is to have a regular meal."

"I don't know," you said reluctantly.

"Besides, I don't want you to get carried away with this notion about reducing your intake of calories and start skipping your meals as well as your snacks. If you skip your meals, you will tend to snack anyway, and there are not too many snacks out there that are equivalent to a healthy breakfast, lunch, or supper. Besides, starving yourself does not work. That's another thing I want to discuss with you—over lunch."

18

A Bit About Crash Diets

We hurried across the next intersection and decided to dodge the snow that was lashing against us by going underground into the concourse. We went through a maze of boutiques and fast food outlets and finally settled for a restaurant close to where you work.

The arrangement inside reminded me of my dad's place back in a small town on the east coast. My mind drifted for awhile before I decided to order a heap of salad and a tuna sandwich.

You were still trying to make up your mind—not on what to order but whether you should order anything at all. It seemed appropriate that I continue from where I left off.

"Your body has a survival mechanism that kicks in when you try to starve yourself. You have genetically inherited the ability to automatically store fat to be used on rainy days. In these abundant times, most of us may not need all that fat, but it is there anyway. The body must maintain a certain percentage of fat which is dictated by your present condition. Under adverse conditions, those percentages go up.

The fat producing survival mechanism will be triggered when we start skipping meals. Not eating when you are hungry is unnatural. Your body knows that it is going to shrivel up if you do this. Your metabolism will slow down to the point where it becomes very difficult to lose more fat. It may not regain its normal rate once you are off your diet, and that is when you will really gain weight. That's why even if you do successfully lose a lot of weight by starving yourself, it will come back.

It is bad enough if you go on a crash diet, but if you are also engaged in an exercising spree, then you are really asking for trouble. How are you going to get the energy to exercise?"

"Maybe that was why I used to struggle," you said when you reflected back on the times when you worked out on an empty stomach.

"If your body cannot get the proper fuel from carbohydrates, your primary source of fuel, then it will have to get it from somewhere else."

"Not from fat?" you asked. You had a strong suspicion that it wasn't but you had to ask anyway.

"No, it doesn't necessarily resort to fat as you might expect, but to protein. But the trouble with burning protein is that your muscles need it. You are actually using your muscles as fuel. If you are exercising excessively, you are burning up muscle at a faster rate than it could be created. That is why a lot of people who 'pump iron' without eating properly fail to gain any definition."

"This is contrary to what I was taught in high school," you recalled. "It reminds me of the quiz they used to give us. If you were stranded on a deserted island with nothing to eat, and you had one last chance to get back to your sinking ship, what would you take if you were given the follow choices: A keg of carbohydrate? A keg of fat? Or a keg of protein? You can't take more than one keg because it's too heavy. You never know when the next rescue patrol will come by, so a common choice would be fat. It burns slow. It will last. It provides more energy. Carbohydrate burns too fast. And protein is not exactly a fuel. It's mainly used to repair and build up the body. It is used as fuel as a last resort when fat and carbohydrate are not present in sufficient quantities, but it doesn't burn as slow as fat."

"It's true that fat would be the next choice in the order of preference. But that is under normal circumstances. When you are starving—self-induced or otherwise—the order changes.

It makes more sense to eat three meals a day that are low in fat and high in carbohydrates as part of your desire to 'slash your weight and trim your abs'. You have to eat if you are going to take part in my program because it involves exercising. When you exercise, the body needs fuel to burn.

Carbohydrates is the preferred fuel. It increases your metabolism. It makes your engine run faster. It's like resorting to a higher octane. In fact, the increase in metabolism, in turn, helps you burn the fat that is stored in your body.

That's an important point to keep in mind. Even if you are not an active person—a couch potato of sorts—you can still burn fat when your intake is high in carbohydrate and low in fat. Your metabolic rate will be higher than the metabolic rate of a person eating a high fat diet. The body converts almost no carbohydrate to fat except in unusual circumstances—like the incident I mentioned about Michael Faulkner or when you are eating way too much carbohydrates when you are inactive.

Carbohydrate is transformed into glucose to be used immediately. Most of it, however, is transformed into another sugar, glycogen, for storage. About 400 calories is stored in the liver to be used by your body. And about 1200 to 1600 is stored in muscle tissues to be used when there is a deficiency in carbohydrate. The amount stored in your muscles can be raised to a few hundred calories more by exercising. What is left is stored as body fat, but it is almost negligible since it is usually burned off to fuel this breakdown.

Your body actually uses a combination of carbohydrate and fat as fuel all the time. What percent of which fuel is used at a given moment depends on how active you are, how fit you are, and what sort of activity you are engaged in.

If you are an active person in general, you will burn more fat than a nonactive person. This is another important point that I want you to note. If you are on a high carbohydrate intake plus being active, you will burn even more fat; and if you are also doing your 5 to 10 minutes a day routine, you are well on your way to 'slash your weight and trim your abs'."

"Is that enough time to trigger my body to resort to my cache of fat as fuel?"

"I know what you are saying. Your body burns glucose when it is involved in short outbursts like a 100 meter dash or running up a flight of stairs. Activities like these are generally regarded as 'anaerobic' activities. Glucose is rapidly burned off as energy. Fat, however, burns slowly and steadily; and it fuels prolonged exercises like hiking, a 5 mile walk, or a 10 mile jog. These are generally termed 'aerobic' activities.

But doing your sit-ups for 5 minutes a day is not exactly an anaerobic activity. It may be in the beginning if you have not done any exercise for a long time and when you give up after 1 or 2 minutes. Once you do your sit-ups regularly and gradually stretch your routine to 5 to 10 minutes a day, the *intensity factor* will force your body to reinterpret it as an aerobic activity."

"It's strange."

"Very," I agreed. "It seems that *duration* is not the only factor which constitutes an aerobic activity. *Intensity* is also an important factor to consider. It is like exposing a piece of paper to the bright sunlight by a window for an extended period of time. It will start to shrivel up. But if you use a magnifying glass to focus the rays of the sun at a specific spot, it will burn immediately. A sit-up is comparable to the latter.

Here's another reason why I suggest that 5 to 10 minutes of exercising is sufficient during your initial phase:

Fat needs oxygen to break down and to be used as fuel. When you exercise excessively, your body will be starving for oxygen; you may end up short of breath, and you may be burning only carbohydrate instead of carbohydrate and fat. If you were always inactive, your body will likely interpret more than 10 minutes of exercising as excessive. If you are huffing and puffing after climbing a flight of stairs from one floor to the next, think of what a 30 minute workout will do to you.

Once you become fit and trim, by all means investigate other forms of exercises. If you want to sculpt other parts of your body besides your abs, it is still unnecessary to spend more than half an hour doing a total workout."

"I always thought that's what you had to do if you wanted to stay in shape."

"Not necessarily."

"In that case…" you commented as you continued to scan over the menu.

19

Is It Necessary To Go All Out When Working Out?

"By selecting only those exercises that have the most impact on your abs—namely, sit-ups—you are getting the best results for your time and effort. You will accomplish in 5 or 10 minutes what someone may not be able to achieve in an hour of strenuous exercising.

I am not saying that you should avoid overall workouts. I am merely pointing out that it can be time consuming if you go all out for hours every day for the sake of 'slashing your weight and trimming your abs'—not to mention that you may not achieve those goals.

Suppose your routine consists of 10 different exercises. And suppose you got to the stage where you can perform 50 of each or 500 'reps' altogether—which is a very respectable number. But what if the majority of them do not have anything to do with changing the shape of your abs? So the question you have to ask yourself is, are you really doing enough 'work' at the right places?

If you only include 50 front 'crunches' as part of your overall routine, then try to do 50 reverse 'crunches'. Feel any difference? Then try some of the variations that impart a heavier load. If you can't, or if you 'feel' it before half time, then you know your answer."

"Why?" you asked.

"When you spread out the 'work' over different areas of your body, you are either developing other muscles besides your abs or your abs are receiving less of a workout compared to my 5 to 10 minutes routine.

You should stick to your initial goal—namely to lose a few pounds of fat. That is what phase one is all about, not building massive muscles; building body mass is another option that comes later.

If you put the cart before the horse, you will not see any results behind layers of fat. When you do not see any results, there is less incentive to exercise. When there is less incentive, you are not motivated. If that happens, you just give up."

"You mentioned earlier that some of your clients are taking part in your sit-up routine and an overall workout at the same time," you recalled. "Could I use that approach to speed things up?"

"You could if you are in shape. It also depends on your commitment, determination, and whether or not you can put in the time. For most people, it's too strenuous at first.

In phase two, you can include your sit-ups with a short exercise program if you wish—preferably one that's less than half an hour in duration.

You still have to remind yourself why you are exercising. Your mission statement during phase one was to 'slash your weight and trim your abs'. If you have made a lot of progress, there is the tendency to sit back and relax your commitment to do your ab exercises. It's like getting close to the finish line. You cannot help easing off a bit. But when you do that, you will also tend to become lazy—both mentally and physically.

To overcome this problem, you have to redefine your mission statement in phase two. Your main objective here is to maintain your slashed weight and trimmed abs.

If you are really into it, you will also include the commitment to gain a set of 'washboard' abs instead of just a set of 'trimmed' abs. Or if you found a sport you enjoy, you might even want to throw in the commitment to become the best tennis player in your region, or the best bowler, or the best...whatever.

But your main concern at this stage is to maintain what you have achieved instead of allowing it to yo-yo up and down. If you cannot stabilize your weight, then everything else does not matter: your well define abs, your tone, your bulk, your ability to excel in sports, et cetera. Once you start with that basic idea, you will find that it's like trying to achieve a new goal; and in a way, you are. Unlike your initial goal, this one is ongoing. So don't throw your charts away yet.

If you look at phase two from this point of view, there are easier ways to stabilize your weight. You do not have to be overly active. Sure, you can jog, bicycle, swim, and resort to your treadmill with a vengeance; but if that is the route you are going to take, you have to keep doing it in order to maintain your weight."

"Why?" you questioned.

"You will tend to develop a big appetite to fuel your rigorous exercise habit. I am not saying that it is incorrect to eat a lot when you are active. Of course, you have to eat to energize yourself. But what I am saying is that it is hard to eat less afterwards once your eating pattern is in an upward spiral. And it may reach an all time high to keep your blast furnace going. You will find that you can maintain your weight only when you continue to participate in those activities.

If you lack sufficient 'afterburn', or the ability to burn enough calories *after* your workout, you can compound this problem. Without sufficient muscle mass, you becomes less efficient in burning fat. The more muscles you have, the more fuel your body needs. But aerobic activities alone do not produce muscles.

It's true that you are burning calories when you are in full swing in your aerobics class, but you burn very little afterwards. If you build muscles, your body becomes a calorie burning machine around the clock. A pound of muscle requires between 30 to 50 calories per day to maintain itself, and that means your metabolic rate will be higher. In fact it can boost your metabolic rate up by as much as 20 times! You also need some muscles not just for weight control, but it is also a good idea to develop some now rather than later. Between the ages of 20 and 70, you are liable to lose about 25% of your muscle mass if you are inactive."

"Why do I need a high 'afterburn'?"

"Because you cannot continue working out at an aerobic rate forever. You got to stop sometimes to take a break, and you don't want to start gaining weight when you do that."

"I think that's what I'm going through," you said after you thought about it.

"When you stop exercising, your metabolism slows down and it's possible to start putting on weight even if your consumption is still the same as before."

"It's not only the same, but my total calories do not exceed the daily limit"

I paused for a moment to reflect on your situation. "How often do you skip lunch?"

"Quite often."

"What about breakfast?"

"I hardly indulge in it."

"Having one meal a day is not going to work," I pointed out.

"But it's a fair size meal."

"Enough to make up for the other meals you skipped?"

"I guess you could say that," you admitted.

"Some people wonder why they gain weight when they don't eat as much as their lean friends. Having one huge meal a day instead of spreading it out could be one of the reasons. It's worse if you have it late in the evening; if your 'afterburn' is not that great in the first place, it will slow down dramatically by the time you go to sleep."

"But my daily calorie intake is less than what's recommended," you argued.

"That's true. But focusing on one heavy meal will cause the pancreas to pump more than the usual dose of insulin into your body. That in turn means more calories are likely to be stored as fat instead of being converted into energy—despite the fact that your total calorie count is acceptable.

And I think you are snacking a lot because of the fact that you often skip breakfast and lunch. The calories from your snacks may not be as high as the meals you skipped, but the fat content is likely to be higher—especially in junk food."

"So what I need to do is to spread out my meals, cut my snacking habit, and include some resistance exercises," you casually concluded.

"I know it's harder to do than it sounds. That's why it's important to continue your sit-up routine at this stage.

The *intensity factor* of your sit-ups still plays an important role in phase two:

1. It's a reminder that sit-ups are resistance exercises as well as aerobic. When you look at sit-ups from this point of view, it tends to encourage you to try other forms of resistance exercises.

2. As in phase one, it also intensifies your thoughts; your objective is to maintain your weight at this stage—and perhaps even to achieve a set of 'washboard abs'. That will remind you to be more selective in what you eat.

3. During periods of inactivity—when you have to take a break—it is easier and more efficient to sacrifice 5 minutes of your busy schedule to sneak in some sit-ups than to try to squeeze in an overall workout. It keeps you in shape and allows you to return to your overall aerobic or resistance activity much easier."

"I should start working out again," you said to yourself.

"Remember, you will lose muscle mass if you just engaged in aerobic activities—or endurance activities as it's also sometimes called—and nothing else. Your muscles can atrophy due to neglect.

In phase one, you have substituted the duration of your routine with its *intensity* to lose weight and trim your abs more effectively. I suggest that in phase two, you add to or substitute some of your endurance types of activities with strength training.

I am not telling you to scrap your aerobic classes, nor am I suggesting that you should start pumping iron to become muscle bound. In fact, those two activities can balance each other by providing tone as well as body mass; you will not become too lean nor too bulky.

An endurance workout can assist in trimming other parts of your body, help set your metabolic pace, provide cardiovascular benefits, and be a lot of fun. It's something I suggest for those whose only means of recreation is to meets regularly every weekend to participate in sedentary activities that encourages incessant nibbling and snacking. I just want to remind you not to be a slave to it. If you can handle a 10 week, 1 hour, 3 times a week schedule, then that's fine. Just don't stretch it to 52 weeks."

"I can't imagine doing that."

"That's just figuratively speaking. But there are people whose routine are just as *intense*."

"Are you saying that you don't recommend an overall routine which is as *intense* as a sit-up routine?"

"Earlier I said that it was OK to add your sit-up routine to your overall exercise program if you can do it. But if you want every muscle in your body to ripple like your abs, you have to subject them to the same level of *intensity*. Then you will be engaging in what I called a *rigorous* activity—as opposed to a *vigorous* one.

There is a difference. A vigorous activity involves a heavy workout—but it is within your threshold of tolerance. A rigorous activity, however, implies that your are pushing your body to the limit and exposing it to wear and tear as well as burning calories. If you run a 30 mile marathon 3 times a week, that is a lot of stress on your knees, hips, and internal organs.

Although building muscles is an efficient way to burn extra calories, you can also overdo it. I know people who force themselves to lift heavy weights for 1 to 1 1/2 hours, 4 or 5 times a week. There are warning signs, but they do not heed them. A lot of internal injuries are not obvious until it is too late. The disks between your spine becomes less flexible as you become older. The same goes with the cartilage between your joints. They can easily collapse if they are subjected to an excessive amount of stress over an extended period of time. You will feel a lot of rubbing when the space between your joints diminishes; and that can be very, very painful.

When I was forced to do something I didn't feel comfortable during the heyday of my rigorous martial arts training, there was often a voice in the back of my mind that used to say, 'Oh no, not again.' I had suppressed that voice back then instead of listening to it. But I was lucky. I had taken lots of breaks, but others were not so lucky. They stuck to it regardlessly, and they suffer all sorts of physical problems.

The trouble with an unyielding workout schedule is that it can also clash with your family and work schedule. A do or die attitude is very noble when it comes to accomplishing a difficult task, but you have to ask yourself if it is worth doing it at the expense of ignoring everyday tasks that require immediate attention. When you force your spouse to play the role that you are supposed to play, then life becomes stressful.

The other option is to subject yourself to an unduly amount of mental and physical stress by 'doing it all'. But then it is like burdening yourself with too much 'load'. Overloading your mental and physical capacity defeats one of the main reasons why you are exercising in the first place: to relieve tension. If you went about it the wrong way in phase one, you are liable to quit. It is just as easy to quit in phase two if you push yourself more than you have to."

"I like the idea of having some control in what I do and when to do it," you confessed.

"It's a good idea to take a break whenever you want to. Sometimes you have to stop what you are doing or skip a class or two out of necessity; at other times, you just want to take a break because of boredom or because you are becoming more active in other areas of your life. These mini breaks here and there will help you ward off any thoughts of quitting.

You will not get much of a break, however, in phase one. I want you to stick it out for a couple of months because my sit-ups also play an important part in reminding you not to indulge in foods that are dripping in fat. Everytime you do your routine, you are not just strengthening your abs, you are also conditioning your mental commitment to achieve the image of the new YOU.

By the time you reach phase two, it's OK to take a short break now and then from your sit-up or from any other types of exercises you may be engaged in; by then you have gained enough discipline to remain committed. You will have more respect for your body when your abs, the most difficult part of your body to trim, is starting to gain washboard status.

For variety, I also suggest that you make use of your normal everyday activities that are comparable to an aerobic or resistance activity. You could take the stairs up two or three floors instead of taking the elevator or park your car away from the madden crowd and walk.

Also, OK, you ready for this???"

"At this point, I think I can take anything you throw at me."

"Try to take part in chores around the house. Tasks like gardening, raking the leaves, lifting the ladder, pushing the wheelbarrow, cutting the grass, cleaning the windows, shovelling snow—careful here, take a break now and then when you have to shovel a lot, help packing and unpacking the groceries, et cetera."

"I take that back," you said with a chuckle.

"And don't ignore the possibility of engaging in an active sport. Your weekly baseball game or your weekly outing at the bowling alley can contribute to your overall workout. My daughter, who is very active, only jogs whenever she feels like it. She's already engaged in enough calorie burning activities from her participation in sports. If you are very active in all walks of life, it makes little sense to slip into your bicycling jersey after work and disappear for a couple of hours. Why do more to maintain your weight if you do not have to?

And don't forget about your physical activities on the job. We can learn a thing or two from people who burn a lot of calories at work: the traffic director who is on his feet all day, the security guard who makes his rounds through a multilevel shopping mall, the police officer whose beat involves a hilly terrain...

Some of them may not look aerobically fit, but their cholesterol level tends to be more impressive than those who are aerobically active because they are eating the right amount of food to fuel the right amount of exercise.

Each of those activities may not burn as many calories as dancing to the rhythm of an exercise program for an hour, but the sum of those activities on a weekly count can easily add up to a substantial amount. Remember, you are performing your everyday activities every day and not just for an hour three times a week. When you think about it in those terms, it contributes a lot towards maintaining your proper weight.

If you are very active at home, at work, and at play, you can still join an endurance or strength training class; but use it to supplement your normal everyday activities and your sit-ups instead of replacing them.

It's interesting to note that I still go all out on my workout during certain months. But I do it for a reason. I still compete. When the time comes for me to train hard, I train hard. This is different from training hard all the time for no reason. And when the tournament is over, I take it easy. I may even stop for awhile.

Professional athletes in every type of sport have rest periods during the off season. Why shouldn't you?"

"Are you saying that we should be selective in our workout once we become active all around?"

"That's a good way of putting it. It's like being selective when you snack, when you place an order in a restaurant, when you buy your groceries, et cetera.

When it comes to working out, you should be selective—not just in what type of exercises you do but also when you do them. In other words, workout at your convenience. For example, I leave my weights lying around at a spot where I can immediately get access to them whenever I want. I don't do them at a specific time. The only routine I do regularly are my sit-ups.

One fixed schedule is enough. You don't want one for the gym, another one for the pool, one for the squash court, et cetera. When your workout becomes less regimented, you are making it fun. It's important to factor that in during phase two if you want to overcome most of the problems that we just talked about."

20

The New (And Improved) You

"When you begin to visualize the type of person that you want to be, then you will start taking steps to become that person. The actual act of taking the first steps is crucial.

I made it as painless as possible by telling you to do only one type of exercise: sit-ups. After you have taken the first step, the process of 'slashing your weight and trimming your abs' becomes easier; once you start doing something, it takes less effort to continue doing it—both physically and mentally.

The first step is hard—especially for those who tried every commercial contraption and food supplement on the market without any results. His or her patience becomes very thin with each disappointment, and he or she will tend give up very easily."

"I think that's why my cousin Jane gave up."

"She has to overcome the usual difficulty of starting something plus the expectation of not benefitting from it once she commits herself.

The only thing I can say to her is that she should try to strengthen her mental as well as her physical commitment. Otherwise, it would be like engaging in strength training with the improper *physical intensity*. If the exercises are too easy, you will not reach your potential development.

When you do your sit-ups everyday, it serves as an important reminder that you are serious about shedding your weight. It will be one of the many things that you will be doing to promote the new YOU.

Always visualize what this new YOU is like. Stick a picture of a set of abs that you admire near where you do your sit-ups if you have to. Look at it before you do your routine. The *intensity* of your sit-ups will imprint the image of the new YOU deeper in your mind. It represents what you want in terms of your affirmation. It will remind you to become mentally as well as physically committed to 'slashing your weight and trimming your abs'. Whenever you stop or do not feel like continuing, look at the picture or read over the steps in the exercise section of your workbook and start the visualization process all over again."

"In Jane's case, it was very hard for her to keep going."

"Well let's put it this way: Once she sees and feels that she is making progress, it will encourage her to continue doing the sit-ups. It will mentally fuel her in the same way that food energizes you physically."

"I feel kind of funny looking at a photo while doing my sit-ups."

"What if I told you that it would help if you also state your affirmation out loud?"

"You got to be kidding."

"A verbal commitment will *intensify* your *intention* even more. When you combine the words which you *hear* with your charts which you can *physically see*, with your visualization which you *see mentally*, and with the *intensity* of your sit-ups which you *feel*, you are actually appealing to the main receptors of your thoughts: audio, visual, and touch.
This new YOU will be etched in your mind even deeper. It will become clear that you are not doing your sit-ups just for the sake of doing them. Like I said earlier, when you believe in yourself, you are kick starting a series of changes both consciously and subconsciously.
At the conscious level, besides continuing your sit-ups, you will begin to do other things that will help you lose weight. They may be small things at first, like buying the right kind of oil to cook your meals, walking an extra few blocks instead of driving, doing your shopping when you are full to avoid the temptation of stocking up on junk food, start

thinking about the bike you will buy with the money you save from not snacking, et cetera. As you become more committed, you may even consider other means of exercising, get back into your favourite sport again, say 'yes' the next time your friend asks you to go for a hike, et cetera.

At the subconscious level, your body's internal function will be altered: your metabolism, your heart beat, your digestive system, the burning of fuel—how it is burned, where it should burn the most, what percentage of fat should be included in this process, et cetera. As long as you keep visualizing this new YOU, it will continue to regulate your body's function *as if you are becoming that person, and in some case, as if you have actually became that person.*

It is like the individual who manages to stay lean regardless of how much he or she eats. His or her metabolism is so high that more than an average amount of fuel is burnt. You can become this person who a lot of overweight people envy—by just thinking that you are like him or her.

It's no big secret. You are altering the way you think. You no longer picture yourself as fat and hopeless in losing weight which, incidentally, is the main reason why you cannot lose weight in the first place. Instead, you are thinking lean and mean. You are reprogramming your subconscious, and that means all the bodily functions that are connected with the subconscious mind will have to comply."

"This is really *intense* stuff. First there's the *intensity* from the sit-ups. Then there's the *intensity* from my *intention*, from my visualization, from the audio and visual aids, and from any short term outcome."

"The greater the *intensity factor*, the faster you will see some positive results."

"And the more short term results I see, the greater the *intensity factor*," you realized.

"It's an ongoing cycle."

"That's it?" you asked after you thought about everything I said up to this point.

"That's it. Now all you have to do is DO IT. Start by taking one last look at your bulging midsection in front of the mirror and say good-bye to it. Happy slashing and trimming!"

Afterword

To sum up, in order to 'slash your weight and trim your abs', you have to:

1. Start immediately. It does not take long. You have to spend at least 5 minutes a day. By doing your sit-ups, you will "feel" better because it will be accompanied by the knowledge (which you have just acquired) that you can change your appearance by doing them.

2. In fact, you will "feel" like a new person. Keep the image of this new YOU intact. That is the individual that you want to become. Express that verbally with your affirmation: "Yes, I intend to slash some weight and trim my abs." By being personal about it, you are also being specific. To take this a step further, find a picture of a set of abs that represents what this new YOU will look like, and hang it up near where you do your sit-ups.

3. Do your sit-ups everyday. You will lose your momentum if you take too many breaks. You want to see some short term results to motivate you and speed up your progress.

4. To add to the *intensity* of your sit-ups, think of the region where your sit-ups target when you do them. When you are doing your front "crunches", for example, concentrates on your upper abs. When you do your reverse "crunches", direct your efforts to your lower abs. And when you do your side sit-ups, focus on your obliques. Forget about exercising other parts of your body in phase one; you are mainly concerned with losing weight (fat) around your midsection at this stage. Resort to other activities only after you've lost some weight (fat).

5. Start increasing the number of sit-ups you do to generate more work.

You will not get proper results if you just do 10 or 15 sit-ups and call it a day. And it may still not do you any good if you do not increase them enough to generate more work. That is, instead of doing a total of 10 or 15 "reps", you may decide to do a grand total of 19 or 20—despite the fact that you are capable of doing more.

6. Another way you can increase the *physical intensity* is to increase the load *internally* or *externally*. It's something for your to consider when you find that you are able to meet your initial repetition and load, and you do not want to boost your "reps" again—even if you are capable of doing them—due to time constraint or boredom (or both),

You can increase the load internally by modifying the way you do them. You can resort to an incline board or attempt the harder variety of sit-ups. Another option is to change the order than you do them and/or to do them in sets.

You can increase the load externally by carrying additional weights like a weight plate, a dumbbell, or a bag of rice when you do your front "crunches". You will find that the remaining sit-ups in your routine will be harder to do; it will be equivalent to carrying an extra load.

7. Another way to increase your repetition is to do your normal routine in the morning and your favourite type during the night.

For example, during the day, you can do 2 sets of 50 sit-ups for your obliques (on each side), 2 sets of 25's for your lower abs, and 2 sets of 25's for your upper abs. (Do them before you go to work—it's a great stress reliever.)

If you like doing your front "crunches", then you can do another 2 or 3 sets at least an hour before you go to sleep. Gradually increase your sets until you come close to the 5 minute mark. Your metabolism will still be high hours later; it's like losing weight while you are sleeping! Do not do your exercises immediately before you sleep.

8. When you increase the load, you are liable to slack off a bit on your repetition. Try to build it up again; otherwise, it might not make much difference as far as your work or total effort is concern.

In other words, total effort or TE is equal to repetition plus load. (TE = R + L). If you go up in R your TE will go up as long as you maintain your L. If you go up in L, your TE will go up as long as your R goes up.

Once you reach a level that enables you to get a good workout, stick to it for awhile. It is like stretching. If you have just gained a higher degree of flexibility, for example, you would want to maintain it for a period of time; you would not think of rushing to the next level. You should not rush your sit-ups either.

9. All your efforts will be in vain if you neglected to cut down on your snacks.

One way to do this is by eating a hearty breakfast, lunch, and supper to reduce your temptation to snack. It is better to have a nourishing meal than to stuff yourself with junk food.

As your progress in your program, try to fine tune your snacking habits with your *intention* to get rid of the *habit* . When you get rid of the habit, you can still snack. The difference is that you are managing it, and that will automatically exert some control during the odd time when you treat yourself.

When you reduce your snacks, do not try to make up for it by increasing the portions on your dinner plate. Never! Never! Never! Your body tends to store more fat from one heavy meal (especially late at night) than from several smaller portions at appropriate intervals.

By gradually reducing your intake of snacks and/or the size of your meal, you will have better control of your hunger. Your hunger pains will not be that great. By ignoring your hunger, you are not dieting in the strict sense. You are trying to avoid overeating; you are not trying to avoid eating altogether.

But when you become more active, by all means eat. Snack away. You have to fuel your increase in activity. But manage it by controlling your fat intake.

Don't use exercise as an excuse to increase your snacking, nibbling, and impulsive eating.

10. And even if you did all the above, you may still be disappointed with your results if you go on a crash diet instead of sticking to three meals a day that are low in fat and high in carbohydrates. A diet will produce a lot of mental and physical stress if you are also engaged in other forms of exercises.

11. Once you see dramatic results (such as losing inches from your waist), consider sculpting other parts of your body by engaging in strength training, aerobics, your favourite sport, or even in everyday tasks (that

promote strength and endurance) to increase you metabolism. But continue to do your sit-ups to add more definition to your abs. The combination of your sit-ups plus other types of physical activities in this phase will allow you to develop rock hard abs or "washboard" abs as it is generally called in fitness parlance.

12. Be patient. Remember, fat burns slowly. A gradual decrease in weight is the only way to go. It is safe, and the results are more permanent.

Notes

Progress Report for the month of ☐

Day	Right Obliques	Left Obliques	Upper Abs	Lower Abs	Total
1					
2					
3					
4					
5					
6					
7					
8					
9					
10					
11					
12					
13					
14					
15					

Progress Report for the month of

16				
17				
18				
19				
20				
21				
22				
23				
24				
25				
26				
27				
28				
29				
30				
Grand Total				

Progress Report for the month of ☐

Day	Right Obliques	Left Obliques	Upper Abs	Lower Abs	Total
1					
2					
3					
4					
5					
6					
7					
8					
9					
10					
11					
12					
13					
14					
15					

Progress Report for the month of

16				
17				
18				
19				
20				
21				
22				
23				
24				
25				
26				
27				
28				
29				
30				
Grand Total				

Other Books By The Same Author:

The Bully Buster Book
ISBN 1-896212-03-4

Your Worst Nightmare
ISBN 1-896212-02-6

Not Just Another Self-Defence Book
ISBN 1-896212-01-8

Available in Canada at:

Hushion House Publishing Ltd.,
36 Northline Road,
Toronto, Ontario M4B 3E2
Phone: 416-285-6100 Fax: 416-285-1777

Available in the United States at:

Associated Publishers Group,
1501 County Hospital Road,
Nashville TN 37218
Phone: 1-800-327-5113 Fax: 615-254-2408

Author's Bio

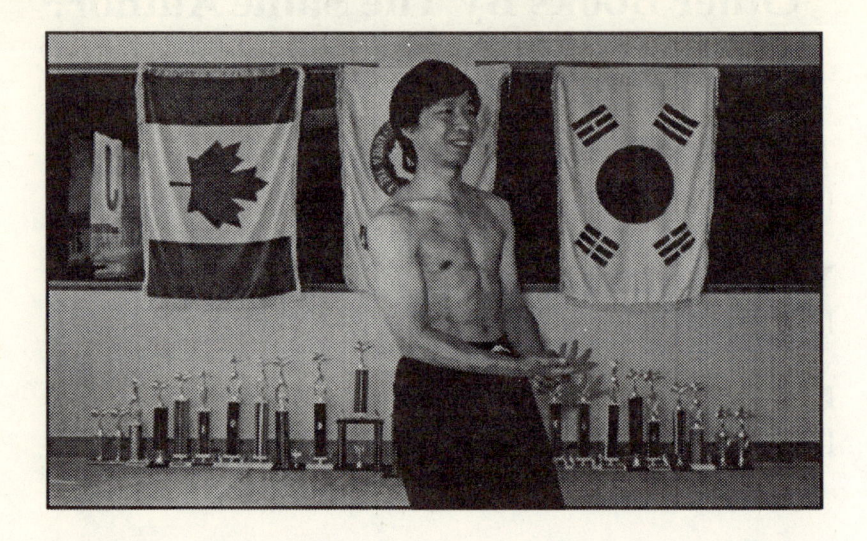

John was born in Glace Bay, Cape Breton, Nova Scotia.

He is not just a martial arts instructor, but he also competes. (He came 2nd in the Canadian Open Kung Fu Championships in 1995 and 1996.)

Participating in tournaments is one of the methods he uses to get publicity for his books. He has to stay fit to remain competitive. He depends on the techniques mentioned in "Slash Your Weight and Trim Your Abs" to give him an extra edge.

This is his fifth "specialty" book. His other books include: "Your Worst Nightmare", "Not Just Another Self-Defence Book", and "The Bully Buster Book". On the back burner, he is working on several manuscripts at once.

When he's not busy pounding away at the keyboard or the heavy bag, he offers motivational, leadership, and stress management seminars to corporations.

He teaches creative writing at York University.